# The Mediterranean Guide to Dessert

Quick and Easy Dessert Recipes to Boost Your Meals and Stay Fit

Raymond Morton

# Table of contents

# Rhubarb Pudding

**Prep time:** 10 minutes I **Cooking time:** 20 minutes I
**Servings:** 6

**Ingredients:**

- 2 cups rhubarb, sliced
- 2 tablespoons maple syrup
- 3 eggs
- 2 tablespoons coconut oil, melted
- 1 cup almond milk
- ½ teaspoon baking powder

**Directions:**

1. In a blender, combine the rhubarb with the oil and maple syrup and pulse well.
2. In a bowl, combine the rhubarb puree with the other ingredients, whisk, divide into 6 ramekins and bake at 350 degrees F for 20 minutes.
3. Serve the pudding cold.

**Nutrition info per serving:** calories 220, fat 12, fiber 3, carbs 7, protein 8

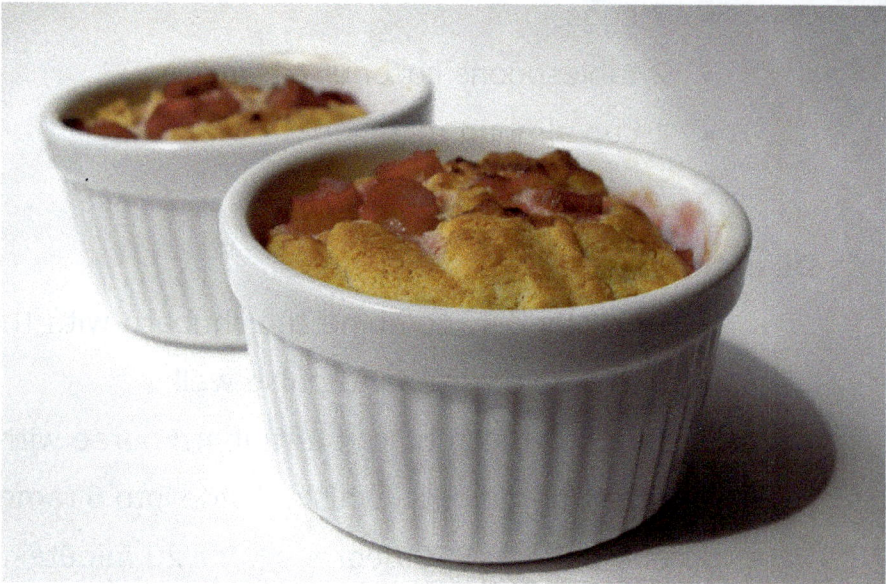

# Pears and Dates Cake

**Prep time:** 10 minutes I **Cooking time:** 30 minutes

I **Servings:** 6

## Ingredients:

- 2 pears, cored, peeled and chopped
- 2 cups coconut flour
- 1 cup dates, pitted
- 2 eggs, whisked
- 1 teaspoon vanilla extract
- 1 teaspoon baking soda
- ½ cup coconut oil, melted
- ½ teaspoon cinnamon powder

## Directions:

1. In a bowl, combine the pears with the flour and the other ingredients, whisk well, pour into a cake pan and bake at 360 degrees F for 30 minutes.
2. Cool down, slice and serve.

**Nutrition info per serving:** calories 160, fat 7, fiber 4, carbs 8, protein 4

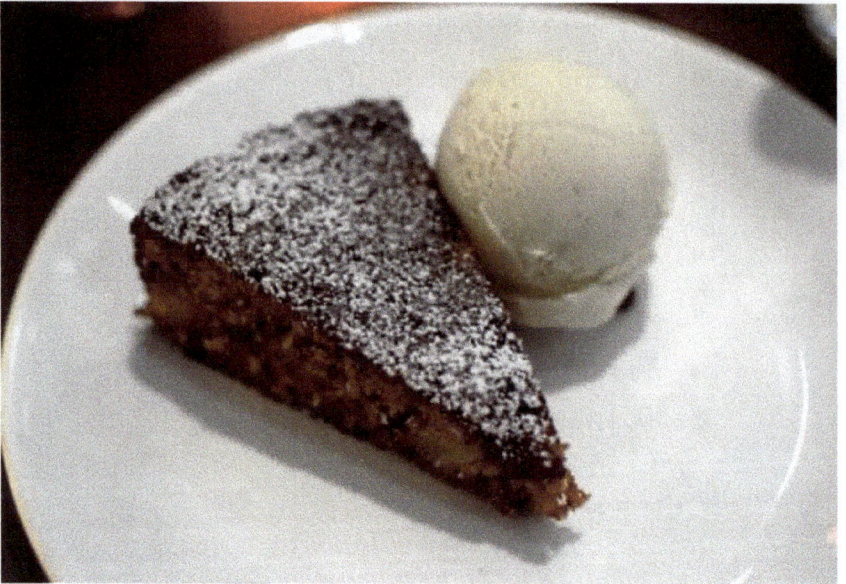

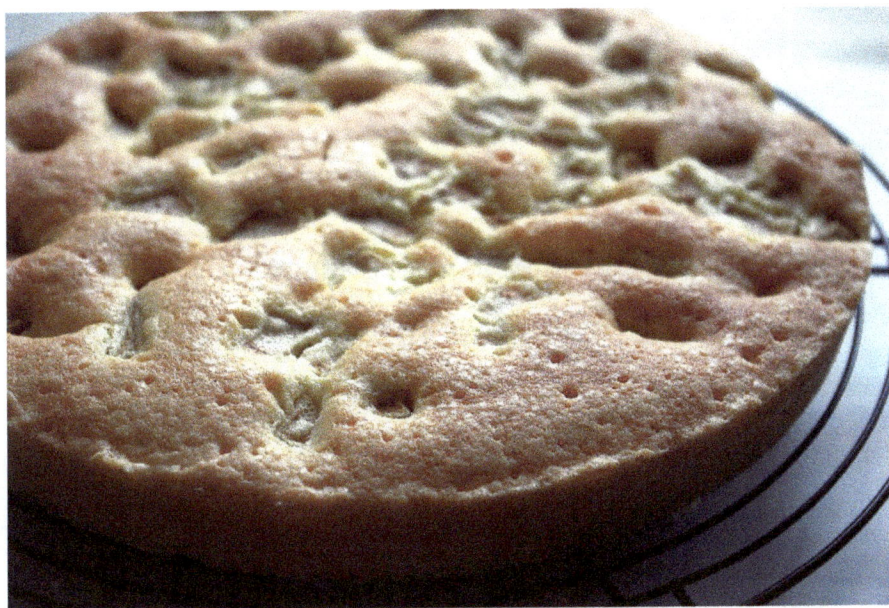

# Pears Cream

**Prep time:** 10 minutes I **Cooking time:** 0 minutes I **Servings:** 4

**Ingredients:**

- 2 teaspoons lime juice
- 1 pound pears, cored, peeled and chopped
- 1 pound strawberries, chopped
- 1 cup coconut cream

**Directions:**

1. In a blender, combine the pears with strawberries and the other ingredients, pulse well, divide into bowls and serve.

**Nutrition info per serving:** calories 100, fat 2, fiber 3, carbs 8, protein 5

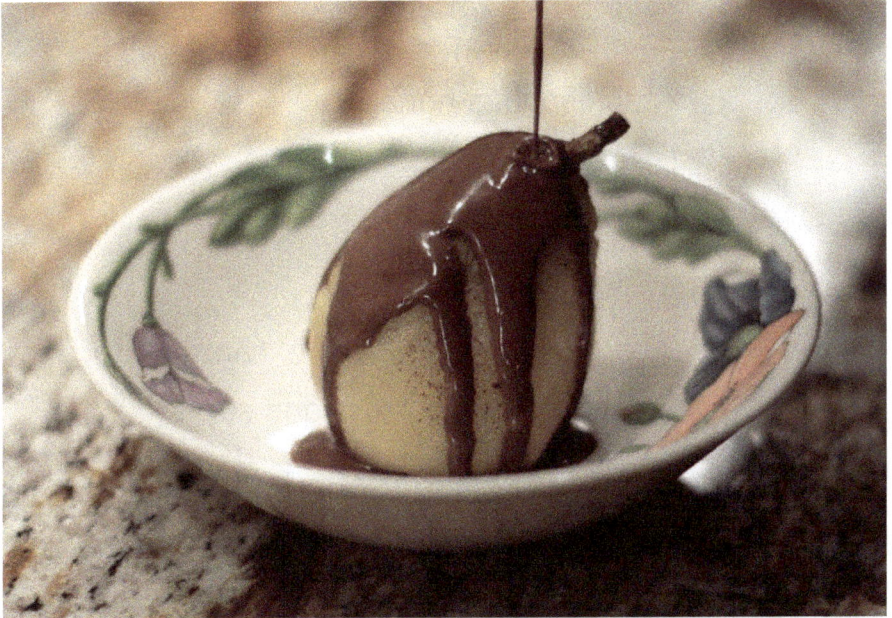

# Cantaloupe Bowls

**Prep time:** 10 minutes I **Cooking time:** 0 minutes I
**Servings:** 4

**Ingredients:**

- 1 cantaloupe, peeled and cubed
- 2 tablespoons honey
- 1 cup orange juice
- 1 teaspoon vanilla extract

**Directions:**

1. In a bowl, combine the cantaloupe and the
   other ingredients, toss and serve.

**Nutrition info per serving:** calories 110, fat 2, fiber 3,
carbs 6, protein 6

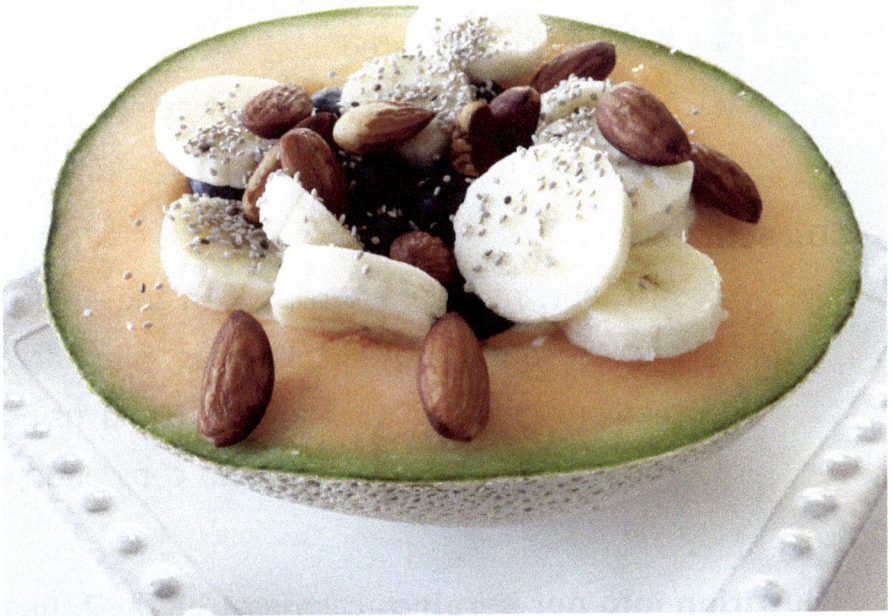

# Lime Cherry Cream

**Prep time:** 10 minutes I **Cooking time:** 15 minutes I
**Servings:** 6

**Ingredients:**

- 1 pound cherries, pitted and chopped
- Juice of 1 lime
- Zest of 1 lime, grated
- 2 tablespoons chicory root powder
- ¼ teaspoon vanilla extract

**Directions:**

1. In a pot, mix the cherries with the lime juice and the other ingredients, toss, simmer over medium heat for 15 minutes, blend using an immersion blender, divide into cups and serve cold.

**Nutrition info per serving:** calories 120, fat 2, fiber 2, carbs 3, protein 6

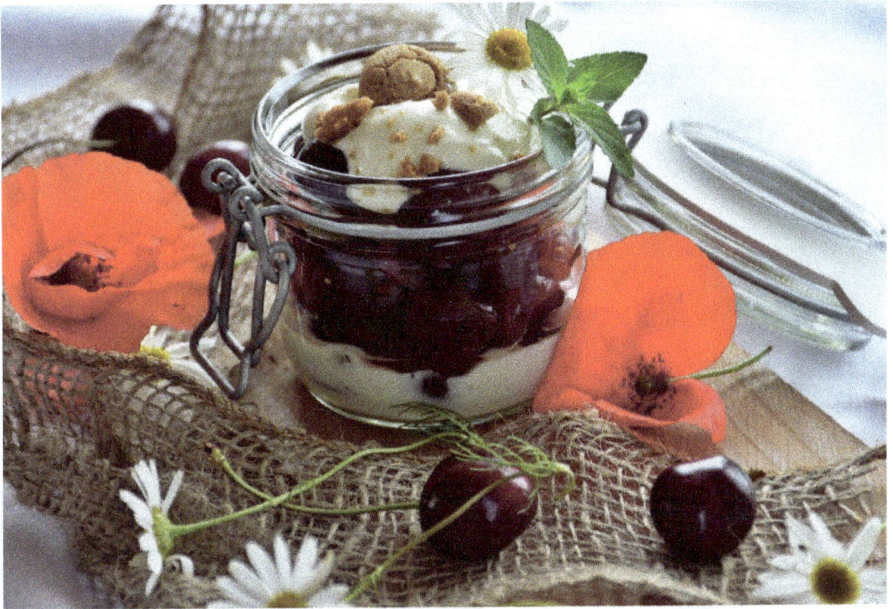

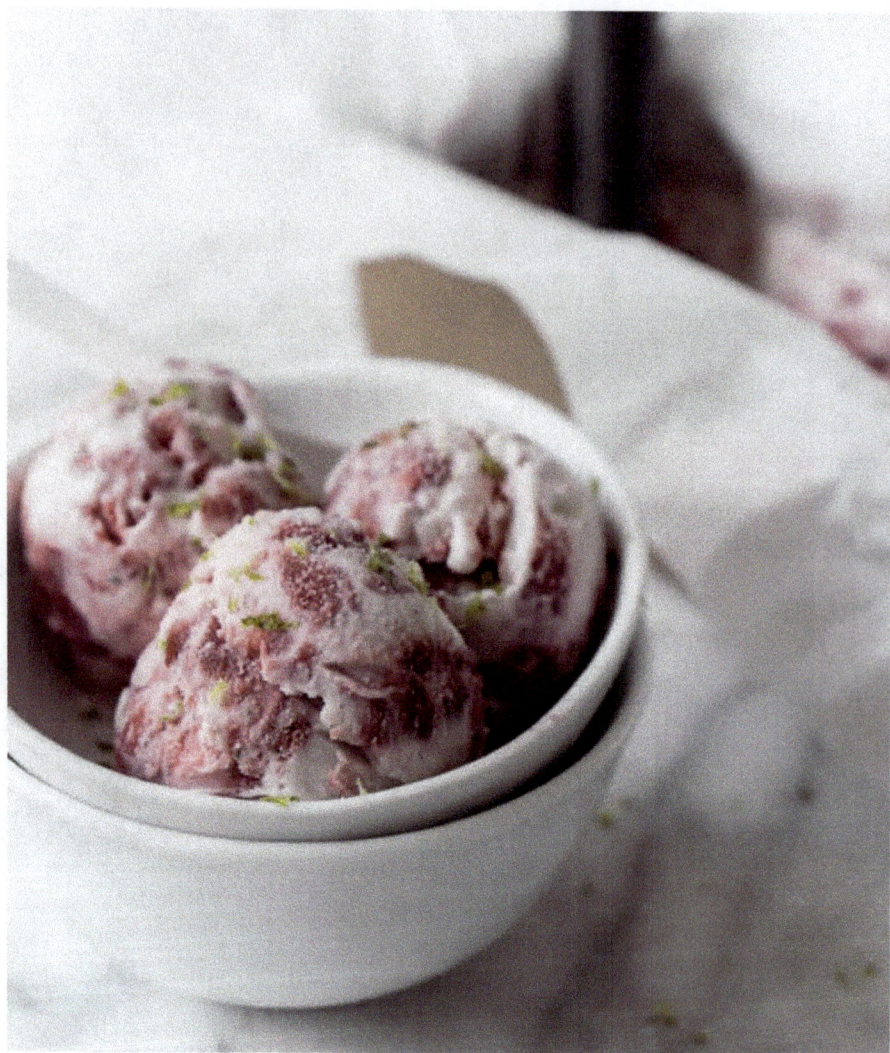

# Apple and Pear Mix

**Prep time:** 10 minutes I **Cooking time:** 20 minutes I
**Servings:** 6

**Ingredients:**

- 3 apples, cored and roughly cut into wedges
- 3 pears, cored and cut into wedges
- 4 tablespoons chicory root powder
- 2 teaspoons cinnamon powder

**Directions:**

1. In a roasting pan, combine the apples with the pears and the other ingredients, toss and cook at 380 degrees F for 20 minutes.
2. Divide the mix between dessert plates and serve.

**Nutrition info per serving:** calories 110, fat 2, fiber 3, carbs 5, protein 5

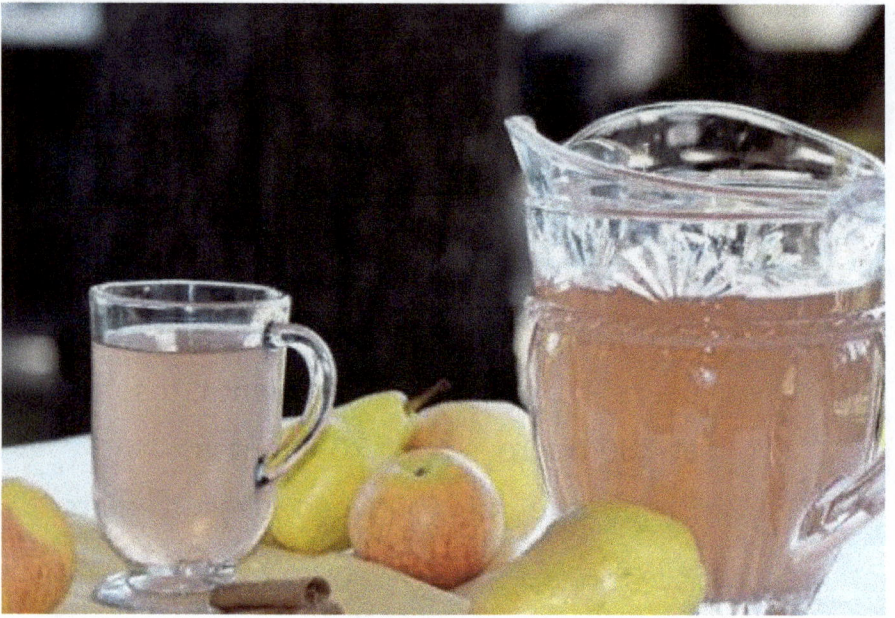

# Ginger Mango Stew

**Prep time:** 10 minutes I **Cooking time:** 20 minutes I
**Servings:** 4

**Ingredients:**

- 2 mangoes, peeled and cubed
- 1 tablespoon ginger, grated
- 1 tablespoon cinnamon powder
- 1 teaspoon vanilla extract
- 1 cup water

**Directions:**

1. In a small pot, combine the mango with the cinnamon and the other ingredients, toss, simmer over medium heat for 20 minutes, divide into bowls and serve.

**Nutrition info per serving:** calories 140, fat 2, fiber 2, carbs 8, protein 9

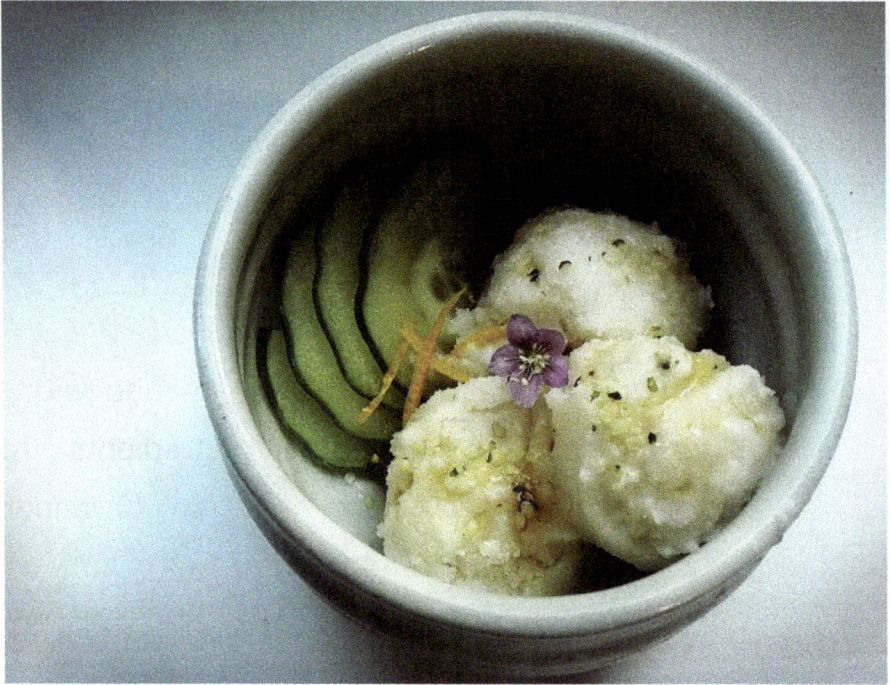

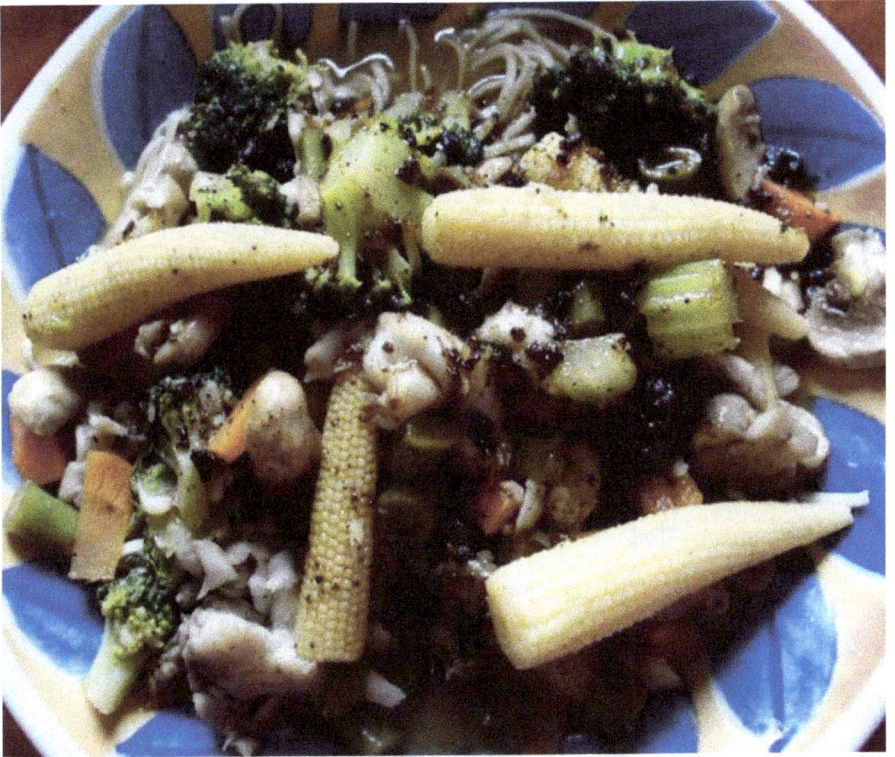

# Lime Melon Curd

**Prep time:** 10 minutes I **Cooking time:** 15 minutes I
**Servings:** 4

**Ingredients:**

- 2 tablespoons lime juice
- 2 cups watermelon, peeled and cubed
- 1 tablespoon chicory root powder
- 2 tablespoons flax meal mixed with 4 tablespoons water

**Directions:**

1. In a small pot, combine the watermelon with the other ingredients, toss, simmer over medium heat for 15 minutes, divide into bowls and serve cold.

**Nutrition info per serving:** calories 161, fat 4, fiber 2, carbs 8, protein 5

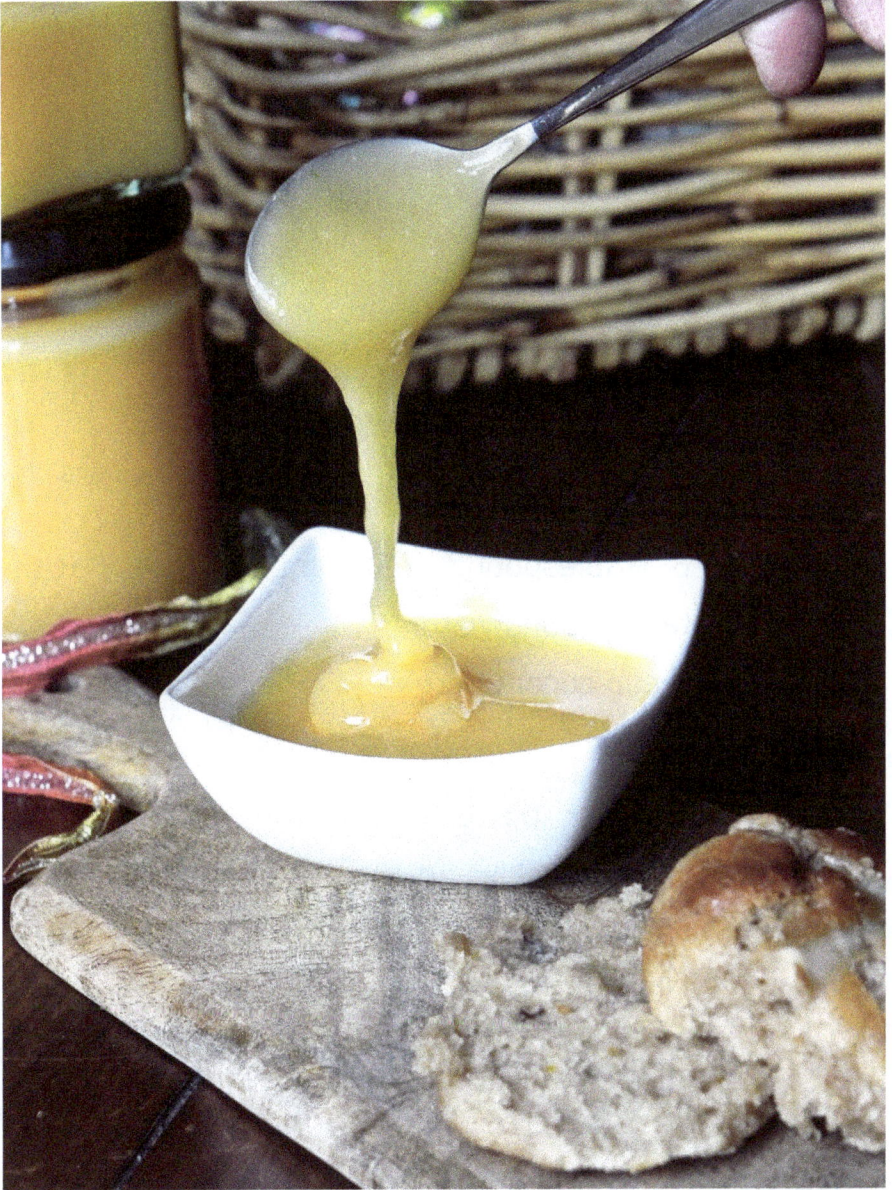

# Coconut Papaya Pudding

**Prep time:** 10 minutes I **Cooking time:** 20 minutes I
**Servings:** 4

**Ingredients:**

- 2 cups coconut milk
- 1 papaya, peeled and chopped
- ½ cup maple syrup
- 3 tablespoons coconut oil, melted
- 3 tablespoons flax meal mixed with 6 tablespoons water
- 1 cup coconut cream

**Directions:**

1. In your blender, mix the papaya with the coconut milk and the other ingredients, pulse well and divide into 4 ramekins.
2. Place the ramekins in a baking dish, add the water to the dish, introduce in the oven, cook at 350 degrees F for 20 minutes and serve cold.

**Nutrition info per serving:** calories 171, fat 5, fiber 2, carbs 6, protein 8

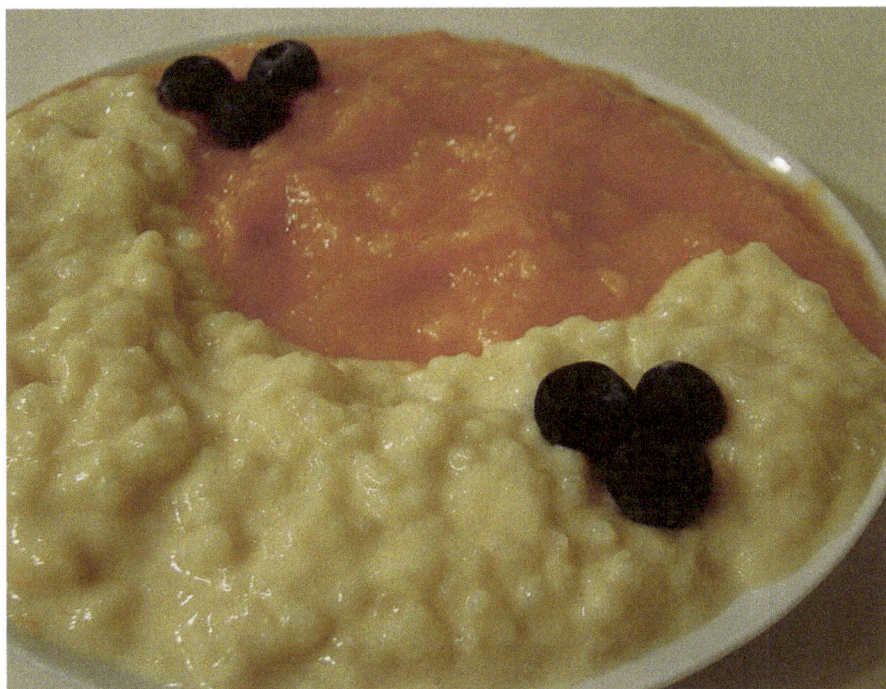

# Grapes and Walnuts Bowls

**Prep time:** 10 minutes I **Cooking time:** 15 minutes I
**Servings:** 4

**Ingredients:**

- 2 cups coconut cream
- 1 cup grapes, halved
- 2 cups rolled oats
- 1 teaspoon vanilla extract
- ½ cup walnuts, chopped

**Directions:**

1. In a small pot, combine the grapes with the cream and the other ingredients, stir, bring to a simmer over medium heat, cook for 15 minutes, divide into bowls and serve cold.

**Nutrition info per serving:** calories 142, fat 3, fiber 3, carbs 7, protein 4

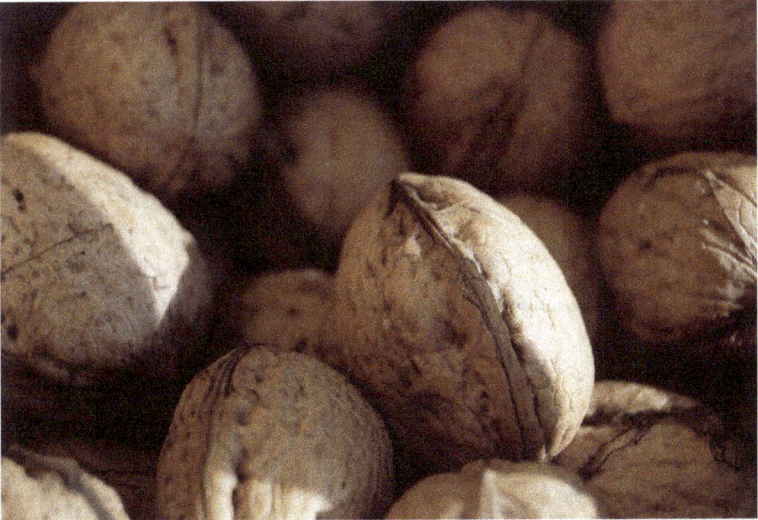

## Papaya Cake

**Prep time:** 10 minutes I **Cooking time:** 35 minutes I
**Servings:** 4

**Ingredients:**

- 2 cups stevia
- 2 cups coconut flour
- 2 cups papaya, peeled and chopped
- 3 eggs, whisked
- 2 teaspoon baking powder
- 1 teaspoon vanilla extract
- 1 teaspoon nutmeg powder

**Directions:**

1. In a bowl, combine the stevia with the flour and the other ingredients, whisk well, pour into a cake pan and cover with tin foil.
2. Introduce in the oven, bake at 350 degrees F for 35 minutes, cool it down, slice and serve.

**Nutrition info per serving:** calories 300, fat 11, fiber 4, carbs 8, protein 4

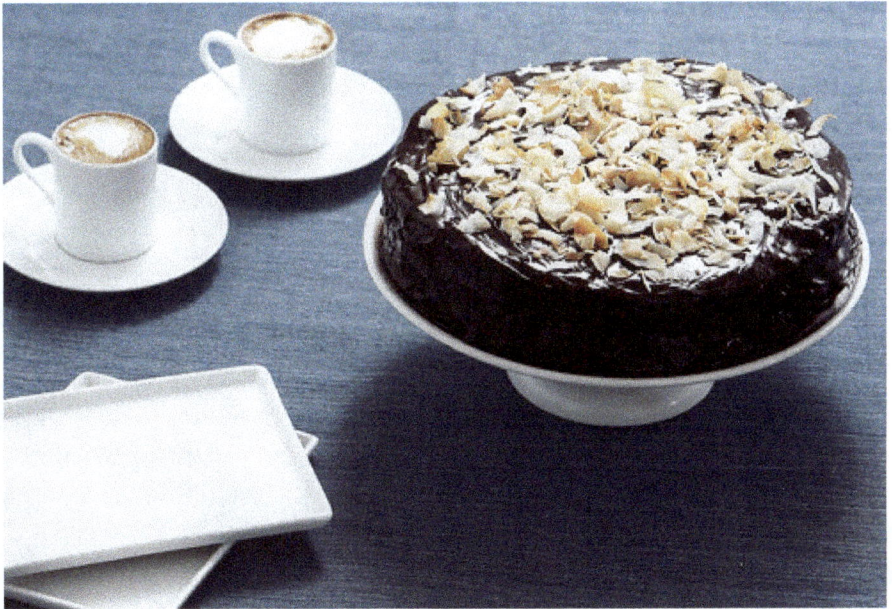

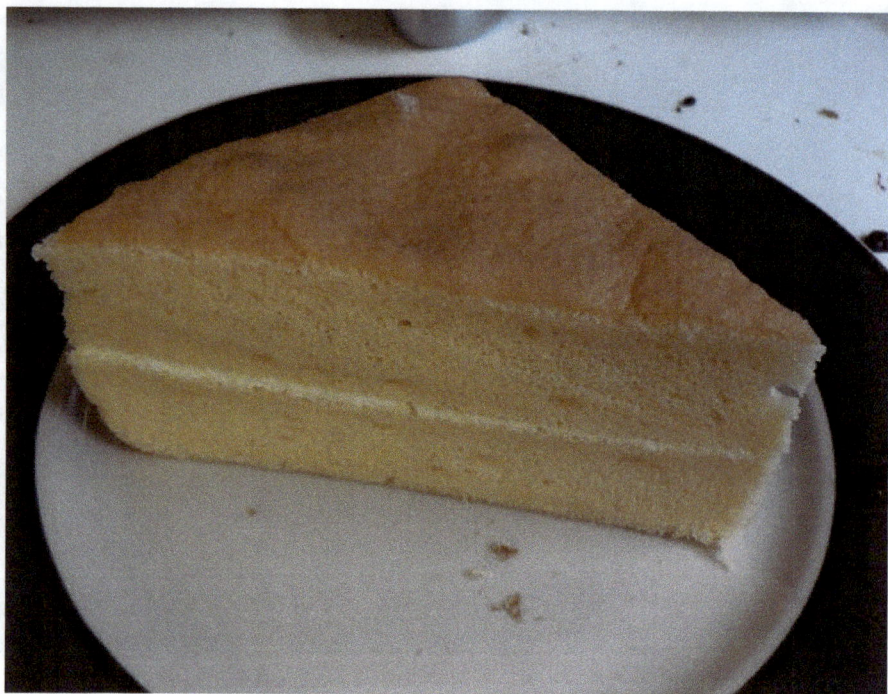

# Quinoa and Blackberry Pudding

**Prep time:** 10 minutes I **Cooking time:** 35 minutes I
**Servings:** 4

**Ingredients:**

- 3 cups almond milk
- 2 tablespoons chicory root powder
- 1 cup quinoa
- 1 cup blackberries
- 1 tablespoon cinnamon powder

**Directions:**

1. In a pot, combine the milk with the quinoa and the other ingredients, toss, bring to a simmer over medium-low heat, cook for 35 minutes, divide into bowls and serve cold.

**Nutrition info per serving:** calories 629, fat 45.7, fiber 9.6, carbs 52.6, protein 10.6

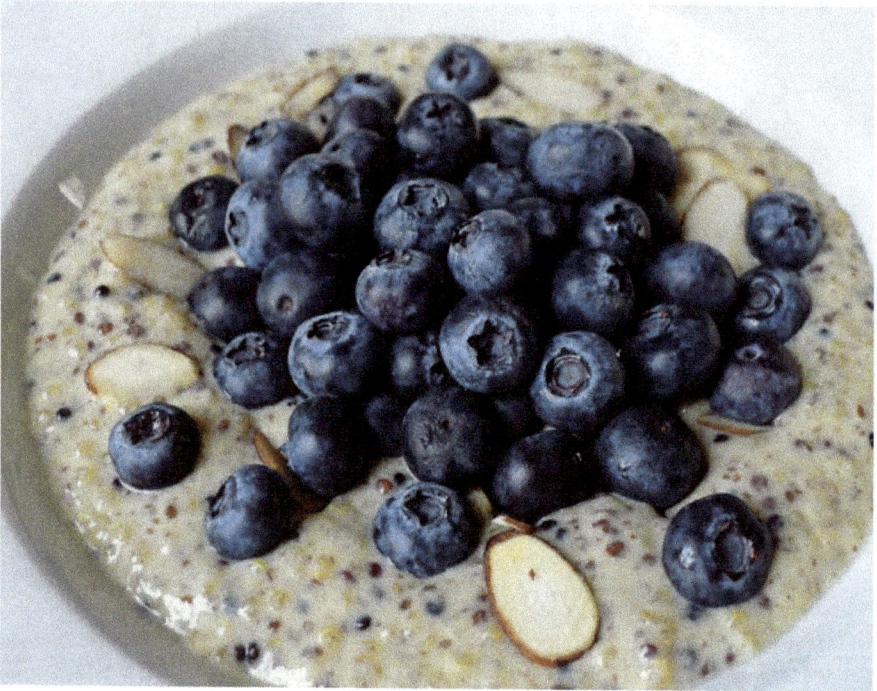

# Brown Rice Pudding

**Prep time:** 10 minutes I **Cooking time:** 30 minutes I
**Servings:** 6

**Ingredients:**

- 1 tablespoon avocado oil
- 1 cup brown rice
- 3 cups almond milk
- 1 cup grapes, chopped
- ½ teaspoon vanilla extract

**Directions:**

1. In a small pot, combine the rice with the almond milk and the other ingredients, stir well, bring to a simmer over medium heat, cook for 30 minutes, divide into bowls and serve cold.

**Nutrition info per serving:** calories 172, fat 4, fiber 1, carbs 14, protein 8

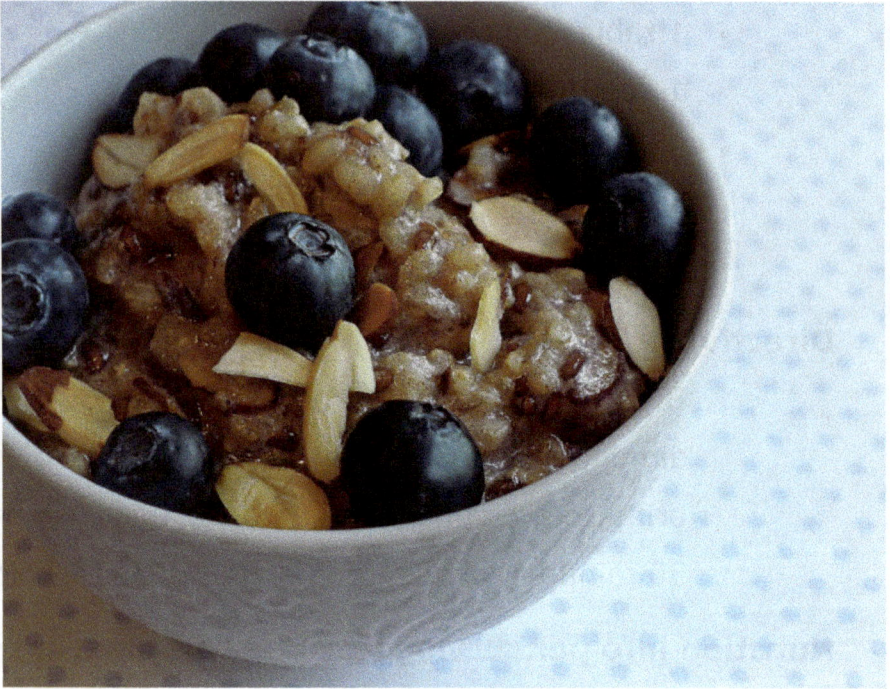

# Peach Compote

**Prep time:** 10 minutes I **Cooking time:** 20 minutes I
**Servings:** 6

**Ingredients:**

- 3 peaches, peeled and roughly cubed
- 2 tablespoons chicory root powder
- 1 teaspoon vanilla extract
- 3 cups water

**Directions:**

1. In a small pot, mix the peaches the other ingredients, stir, bring to a simmer over medium heat, cook for 20 minutes, divide into cups and serve cold.

**Nutrition info per serving:** calories 122, fat 4, fiber 2, carbs 8, protein 2

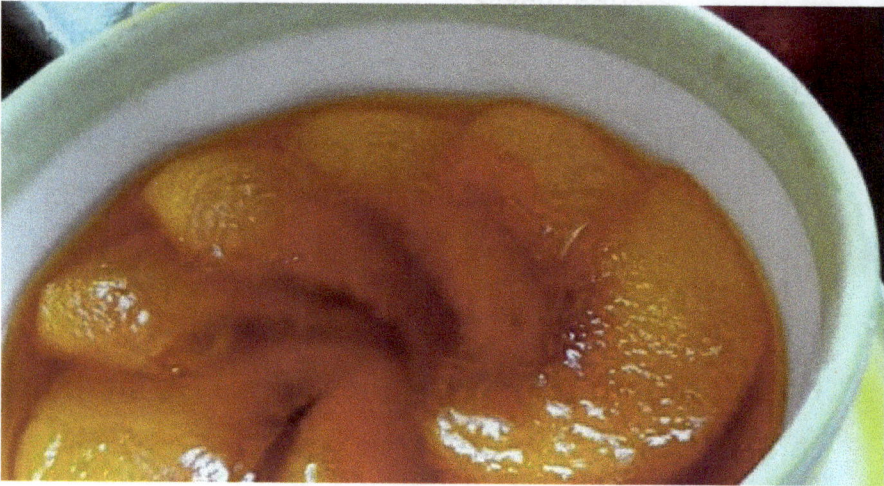

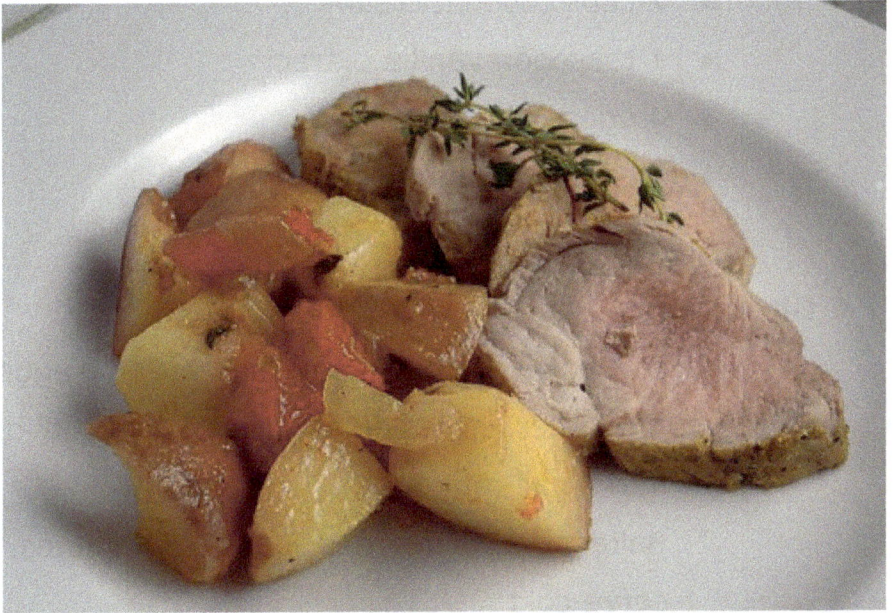

# Eggs Pudding

**Prep time:** 10 minutes I **Cooking time:** 25 minutes I
**Servings:** 6

**Ingredients:**

- 2 cups coconut cream
- 1 teaspoon vanilla extract
- 4 eggs, whisked
- 1 teaspoon lime juice
- ½ teaspoon nutmeg powder

**Directions:**

1. In a bowl, combine the cream with the eggs and the other ingredients, whisk well, and divide into small ramekins.
2. Bake at 350 degrees F for 25 minutes, and serve cold

**Nutrition info per serving:** calories 200, fat 5, fiber 2, carbs 8, protein 8

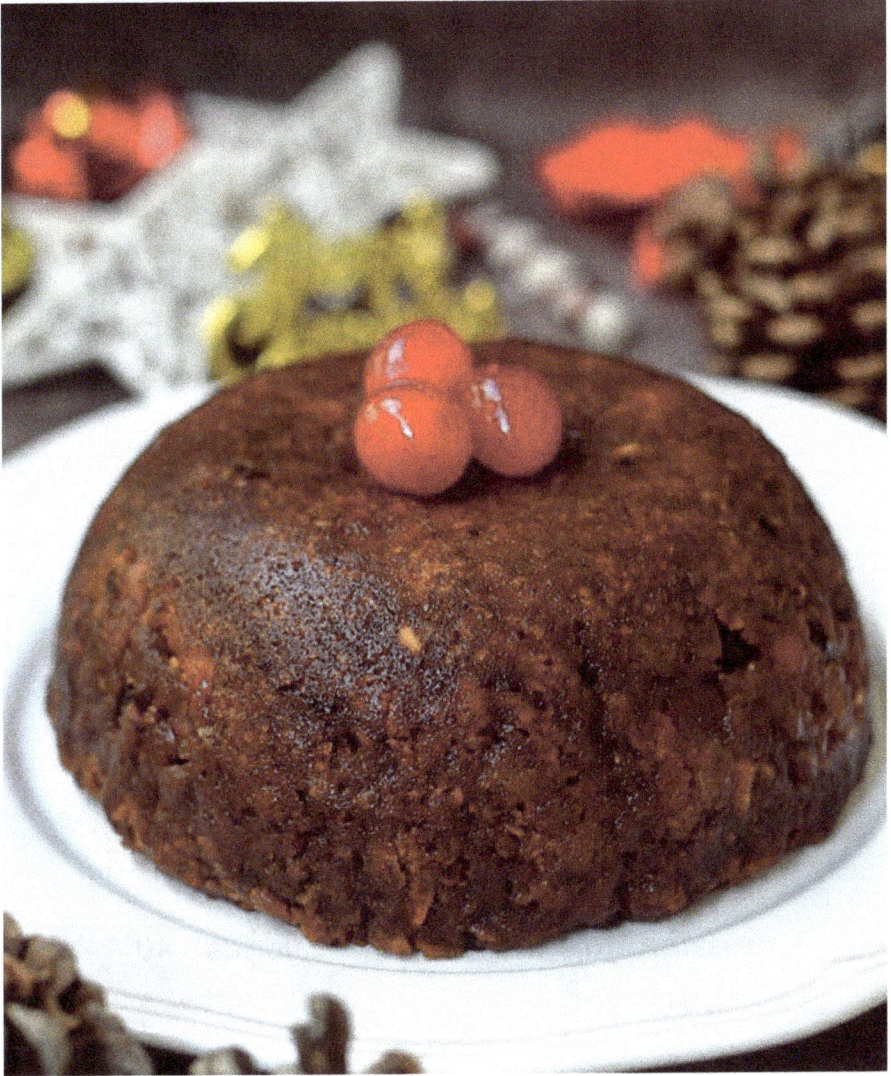

# Apricot Cream

**Prep time:** 10 minutes I **Cooking time:** 0 minutes I
**Servings:** 4

**Ingredients:**

- 12 ounces apricots, chopped
- 2 tablespoons chia seeds
- 2 cups coconut cream
- 2 avocados, peeled, pitted and cubed
- 2 tablespoons maple syrup
- 2 tablespoons brown sugar
- 1 tablespoon vanilla extract

**Directions:**

1. In a blender, combine the apricots with the chia seeds and the other ingredients, pulse well, divide into bowls and serve really cold.

**Nutrition info per serving:** calories 140, fat 2, fiber 2, carbs 10, protein 7

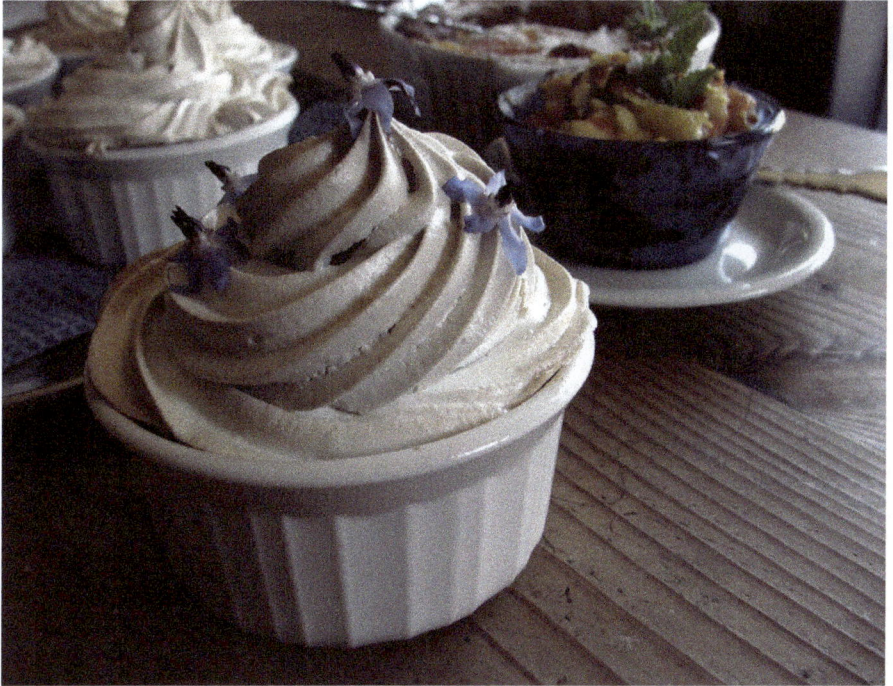

## Strawberry Compote

**Prep time:** 10 minutes I **Cooking time:** 20 minutes I
**Servings:** 4

**Ingredients:**

- 2 cups strawberries, halved
- 2 cups water
- 2 tablespoons coconut sugar
- 1 tablespoon lime juice
- ½ teaspoon vanilla extract

**Directions:**

1. In a pan, combine the strawberries with the water and the other ingredients, toss, bring to a simmer and cook over medium heat for 20 minutes.
2. Divide the mix into bowls and serve cold.

**Nutrition info per serving:** calories 200, fat 2, fiber 3, carbs 5, protein 10

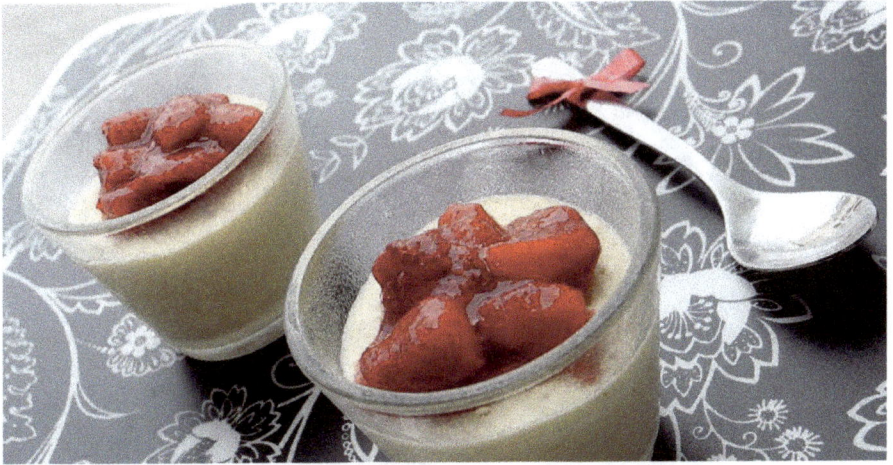

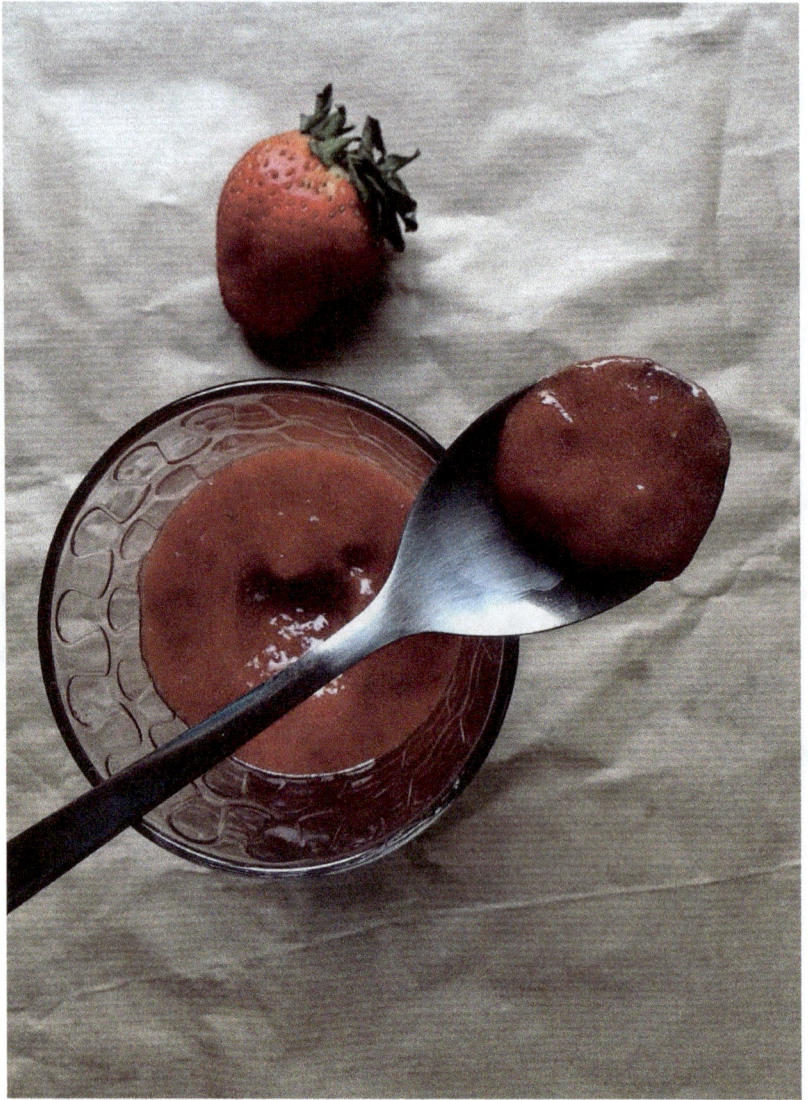

# Honey Egg Curd

**Prep time:** 10 minutes I **Cooking time:** 10 minutes I
**Servings:** 4

**Ingredients:**

- 2 cups blackberries
- ¼ cup lime juice
- 2 tablespoons honey
- 2 teaspoons lime zest, grated
- 4 tablespoons coconut oil, melted
- 3 egg yolks, whisked

**Directions:**

1. Heat up a small pan over medium heat, add the berries and lime juice, stir, bring to a simmer, cook for 5 minutes, strain this into a heatproof bowl and mash a bit.
2. Put some water into a pan, bring to a simmer over medium heat, add the bowl with the berries on top, also add the rest of the ingredients, stir well, cook for 5 minutes more, divide into small cups and serve cold.

**Nutrition info per serving:** calories 140, fat 3, fiber 3, carbs 6, protein 8

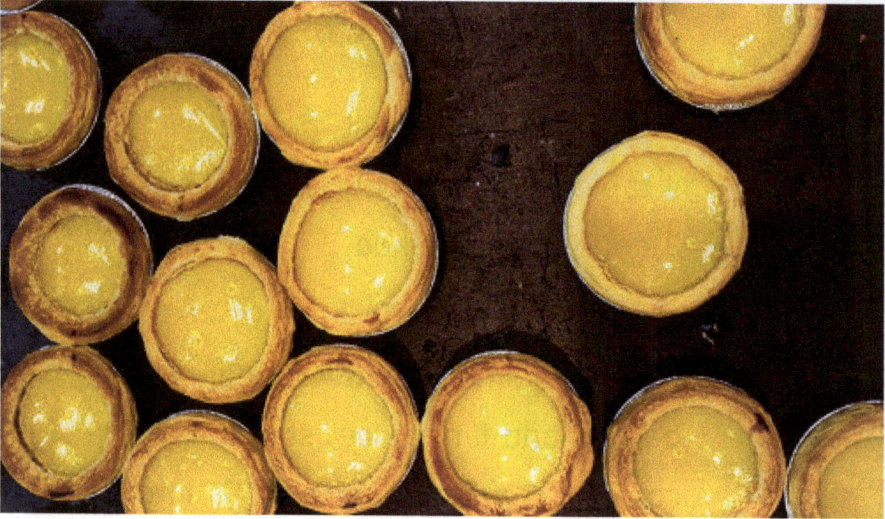

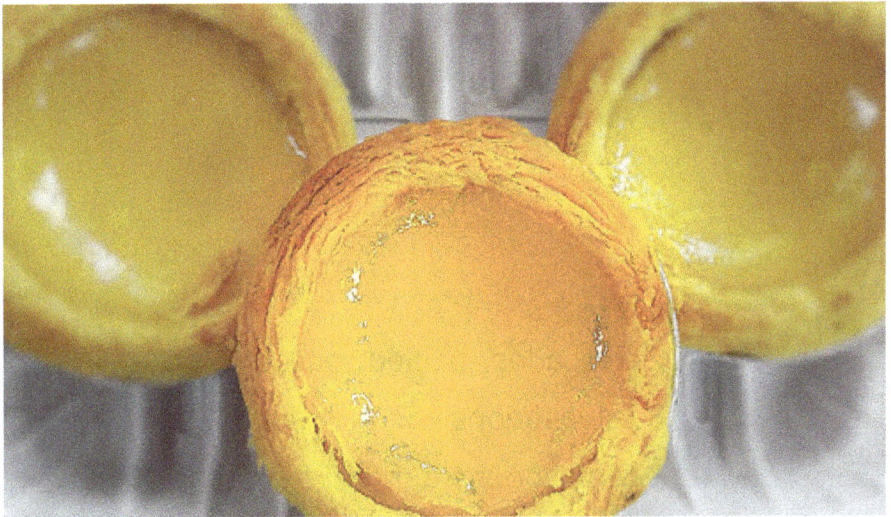

# Coconut Avocado Pie

**Prep time:** 30 minutes I **Cooking time:** 40 minutes I
**Servings:** 8

## Ingredients:

- 2 cups coconut flour
- 6 tablespoons coconut butter
- 5 tablespoons water

*For the filling:*

- 2 avocados, peeled, pitted and cubed
- 3 tablespoons coconut sugar
- 3 tablespoons almond flour
- ½ teaspoon vanilla extract
- 2 eggs, whisked
- 1 tablespoon avocado oil
- 2 tablespoons coconut milk

**Directions:**

1. In a bowl, mix the coconut flour with the coconut butter and the water, stir until you obtain a firm dough, transfer the dough to a floured working surface, knead it, shape a flattened disk, wrap in plastic, keep in the fridge for 30 minutes, roll a circle and arrange in a pie pan.

2. In a bowl, mix the avocados with the sugar and the other ingredients for the filling, stir well, pour into the pie pan, introduce in the oven at 370 degrees F, bake for 40 minutes, cut and serve.

**Nutrition info per serving::** calories 200, fat 6.3, fiber 3, carbs 11.6, protein 9

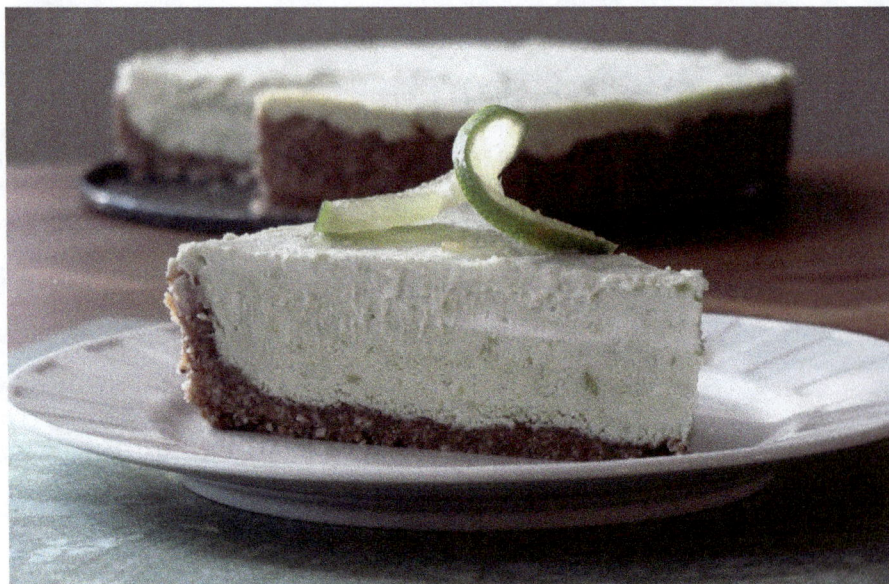

# Coconut Carrot Cake

**Prep time:** 10 minutes I **Cooking time:** 35 minutes I
**Servings:** 6

**Ingredients:**

- 2 cups coconut milk
- ½ cup coconut oil, melted
- Chicory root powder to the taste
- 4 eggs, whisked
- 2 carrots, grated
- 2 teaspoons vanilla extract
- 2 cups almond flour
- 1 teaspoon baking soda

**Directions:**

1. In a bowl, combine the milk with the coconut oil and the other ingredients, stir well, pour into a cake pan, bake in the oven at 350 degrees F 35 minutes, slice, divide between plates and serve.

**Nutrition info per serving:** calories 170, fat 4, fiber 5, carbs 6, protein 2

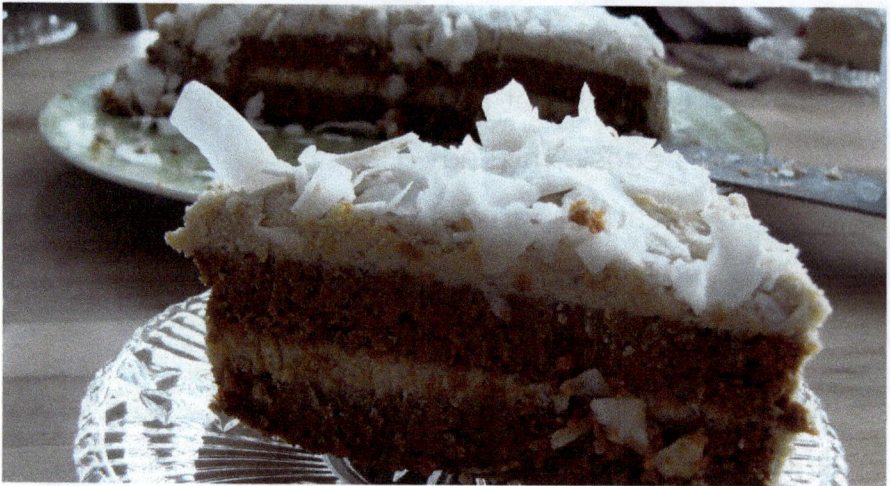

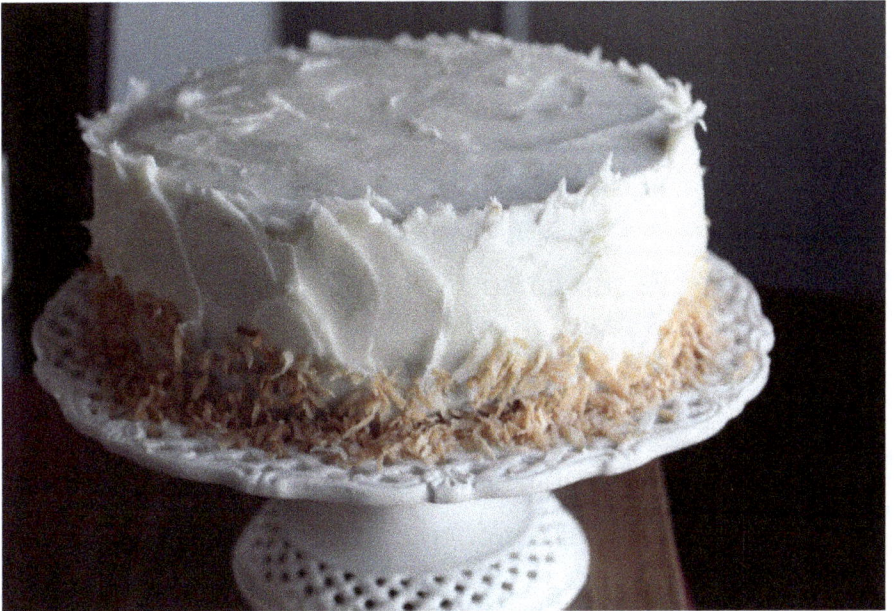

# Quinoa and Carrot Pudding

**Prep time:** 5 minutes I **Cooking time:** 20 minutes I
**Servings:** 4

**Ingredients:**

- 1 cup quinoa
- 2 cups almond milk
- 3 tablespoons coconut butter
- ¼ cup almonds, chopped
- ½ cup carrots, peeled and grated

**Directions:**

1. In a pot, combine the quinoa with the almond milk and the other ingredients, bring to a simmer and cook over medium heat for 20 minutes.
2. Divide into bowls and serve cold.

**Nutrition info per serving:** calories 176, fat 6.4, fiber 5, carbs 9, protein 8

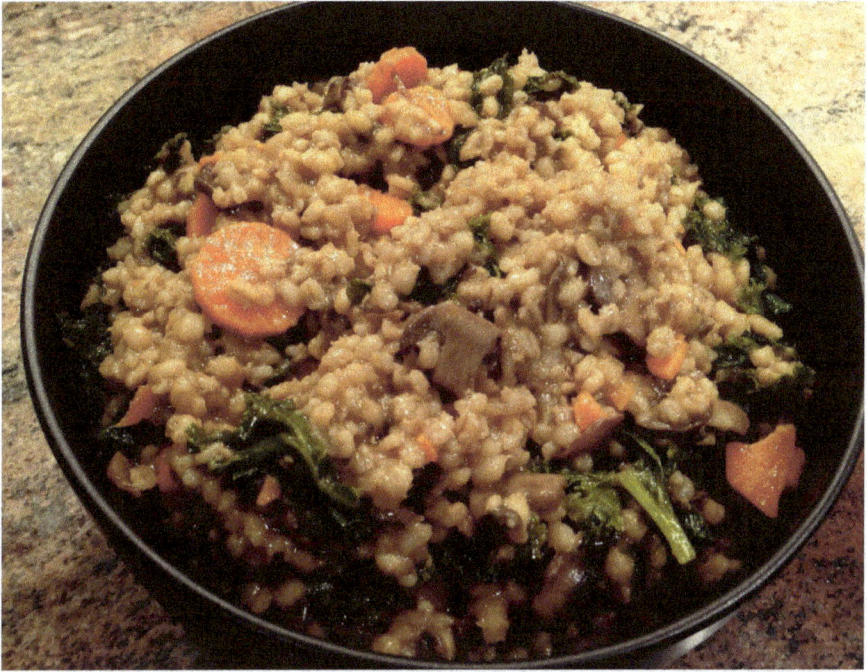

# Banana and Papaya Salad

**Prep time:** 10 minutes I **Cooking time:** 0 minutes I **Servings:** 4

**Ingredients:**

- 4 bananas, peeled and chopped
- 2 cups papaya, peeled and cubed
- Juice of 1 lime
- 1 tablespoon avocado oil

**Directions:**

1. In a bowl, combine the bananas with the papaya and the other ingredients, toss and serve.

**Nutrition info per serving:** calories 370, fat 7, fiber 5, carbs 11, protein 8

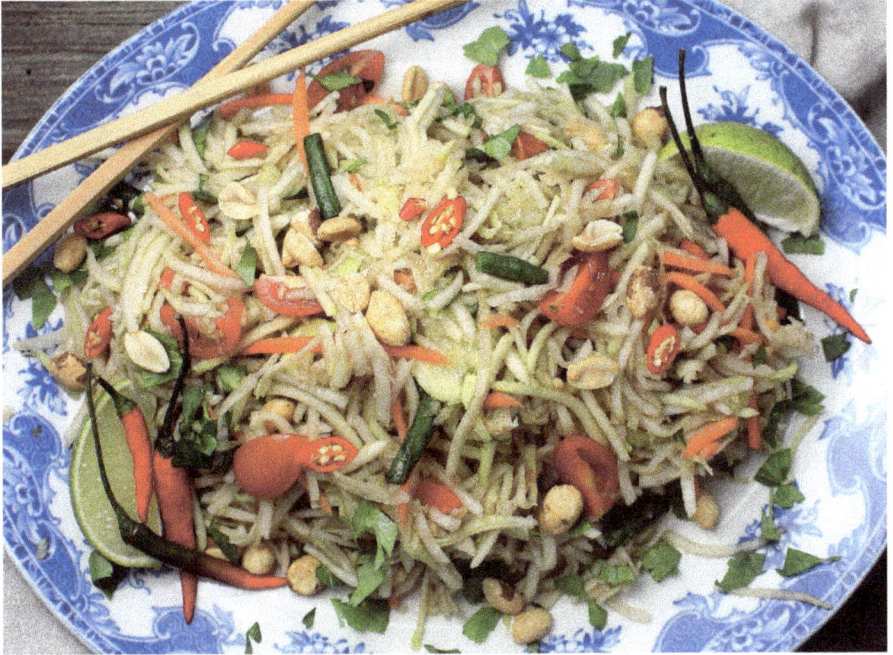

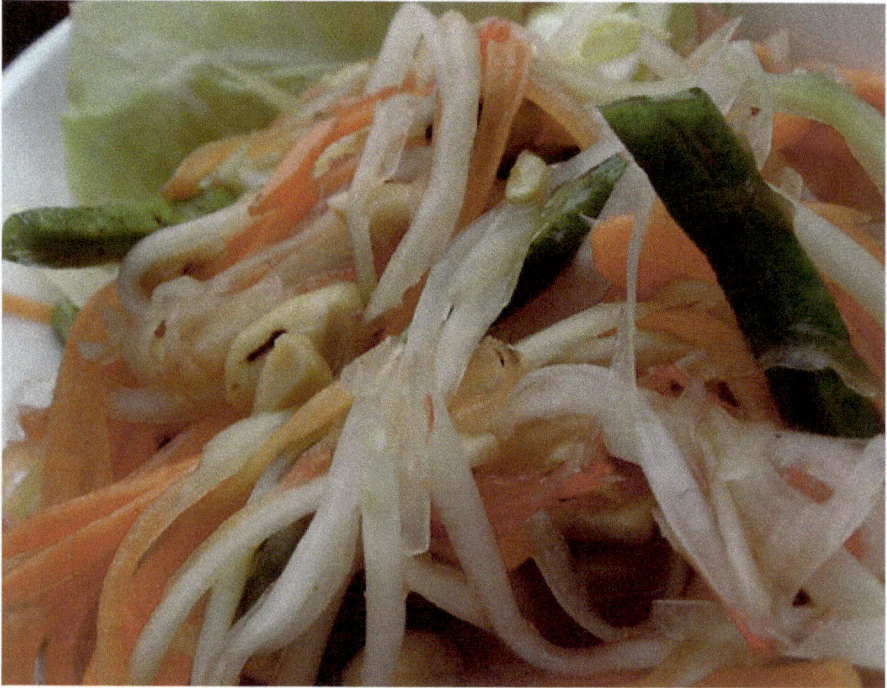

# Honey Orange Mix

**Prep time:** 10 minutes I **Cooking time:** 0 minutes I
**Servings:** 2

**Ingredients:**

- 2 tablespoons raw honey
- 2 oranges, peeled, and cut into medium segments
- 1 cup coconut cream
- 1 tablespoon mint leaves, chopped

**Directions:**

1. In a bowl, combine the oranges with the cream and the other ingredients, toss, divide into small bowls and serve.

**Nutrition info per serving:** calories 150, fat 2, fiber 5, carbs 10, protein 11

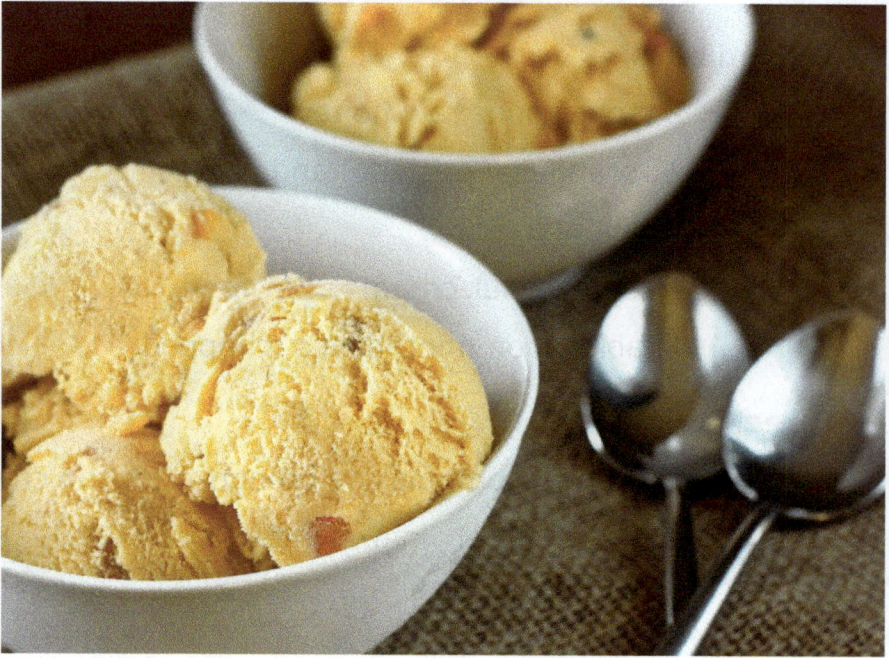

# Green Tea Pudding

**Prep time:** 10 minutes I **Cooking time:** 15 minutes I
**Servings:** 4

**Ingredients:**

- 3 cups almond milk
- ½ cup coconut cream
- 2 tablespoons green tea powder
- 1 teaspoon vanilla extract
- 3 tablespoons chicory root powder

**Directions:**

1. In a pot, combine the almond milk with the cream and the other ingredients, whisk, bring to a simmer and cook over medium heat for 15 minutes.
2. Divide the mix into bowls and serve.

**Nutrition info per serving:** calories 220, fat 3, fiber 3, carbs 7, protein 5

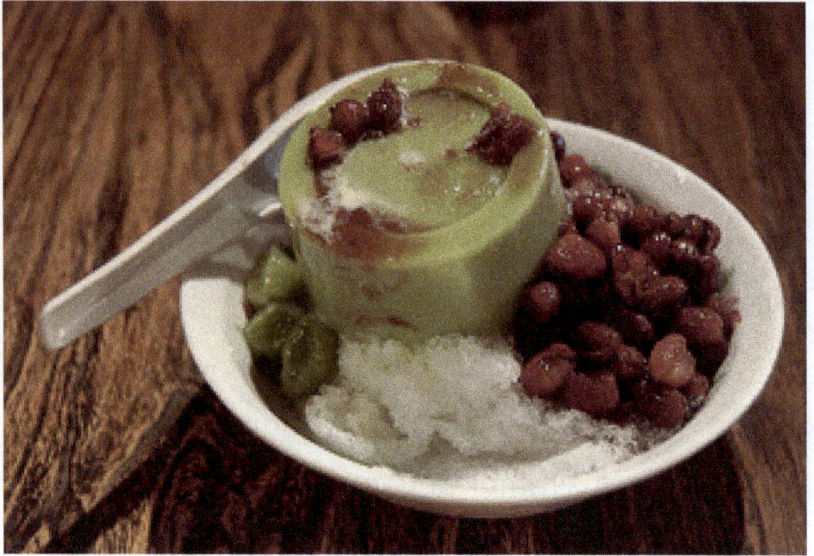

# Pineapple Cream

**Prep time:** 5 minutes I **Cooking time:** 0 minutes I
**Servings:** 4

**Ingredients:**

- 1 cup pineapple, peeled and cubed
- 1 tablespoon coconut oil, melted
- ¾ cup coconut cream
- 2 tablespoons maple syrup

**Directions:**

1. In your blender, combine the berries with the pineapple and the other ingredients, pulse well, divide into bowls and serve cold.

**Nutrition info per serving:** calories 120, fat 3, fiber 3, carbs 6, protein 8

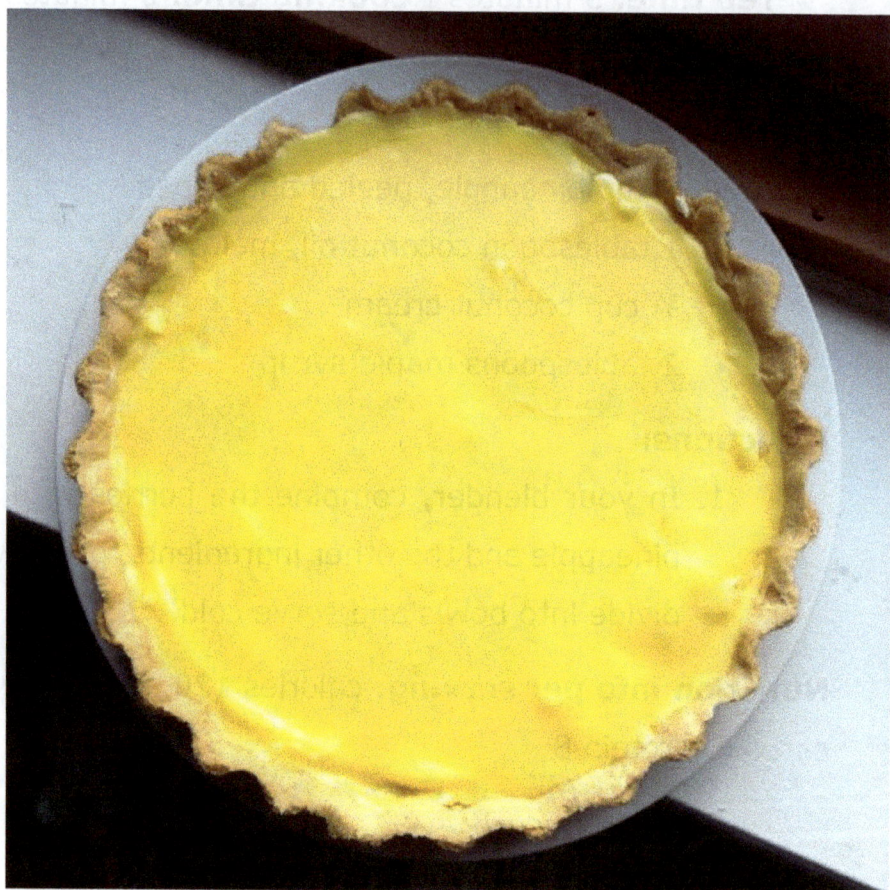

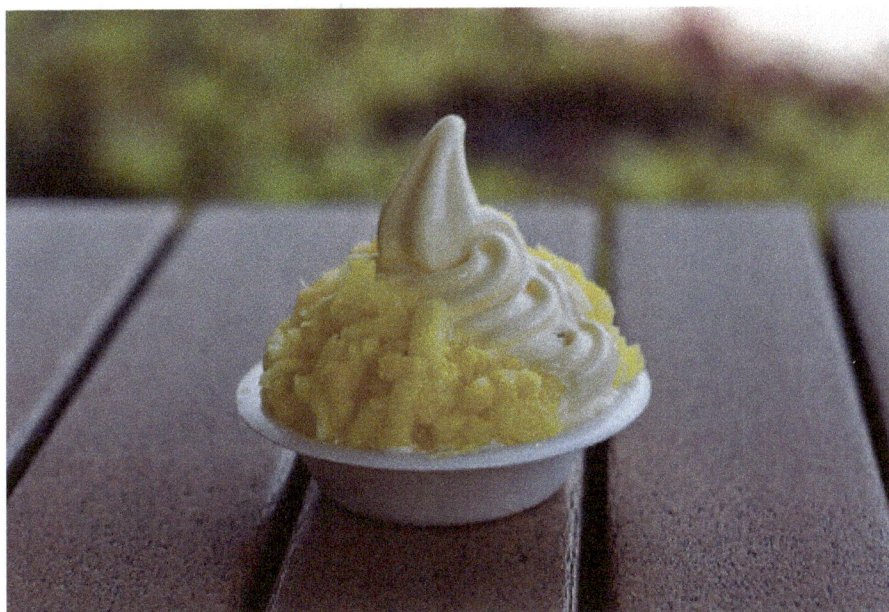

# Strawberries Pudding

**Prep time:** 10 minutes I **Cooking time:** 25 minutes I
**Servings:** 4

**Ingredients:**

- 2 cups almond milk
- 1 cup black rice
- ½ cup strawberries
- 2 tablespoons sugar
- 1 teaspoon cinnamon powder

**Directions:**

1. Heat up a pan with the milk over medium heat, add the rice and the other ingredients, cook for 25 minutes stirring often, divide into bowls and serve cold.

**Nutrition info per serving:** calories 130, fat 1, fiber 3, carbs 4, protein 2

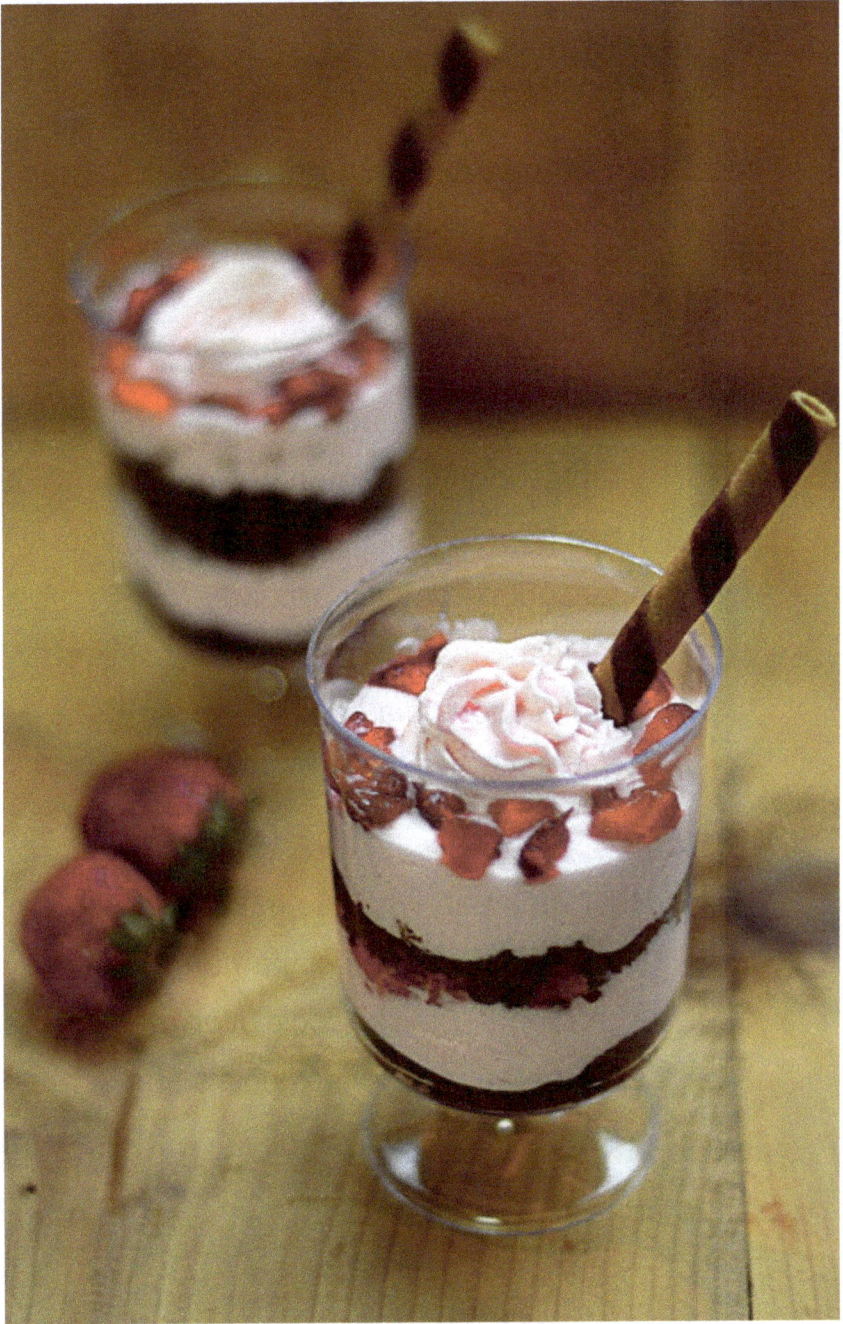

# Spiced Pudding

**Prep time:** 10 minutes I **Cooking time:** 12 minutes I
**Servings:** 4

**Ingredients:**

- 2 cups almond milk
- ½ cup coconut, unsweetened and shredded
- 1 tablespoon cinnamon powder
- 1 teaspoon allspice, ground
- 2 teaspoons ginger, ground
- 2 tablespoons pumpkin seeds
- 1 tablespoon chia seeds
- 1 teaspoon green tea powder

**Directions:**

1. Heat up a pan with the milk over medium heat, add the coconut, cinnamon and the other ingredients, whisk, cook over medium heat for 12 minutes, divide into bowls and serve cold.

**Nutrition info per serving:** calories 150, fat 4, fiber 2, carbs 6, protein 3

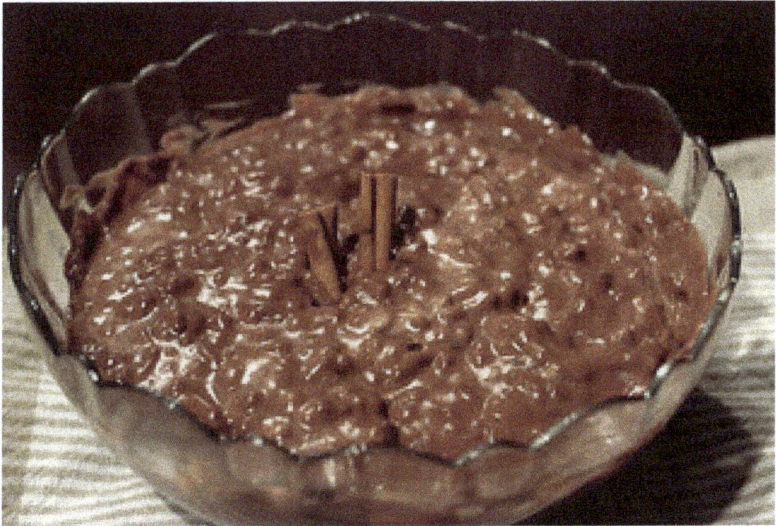

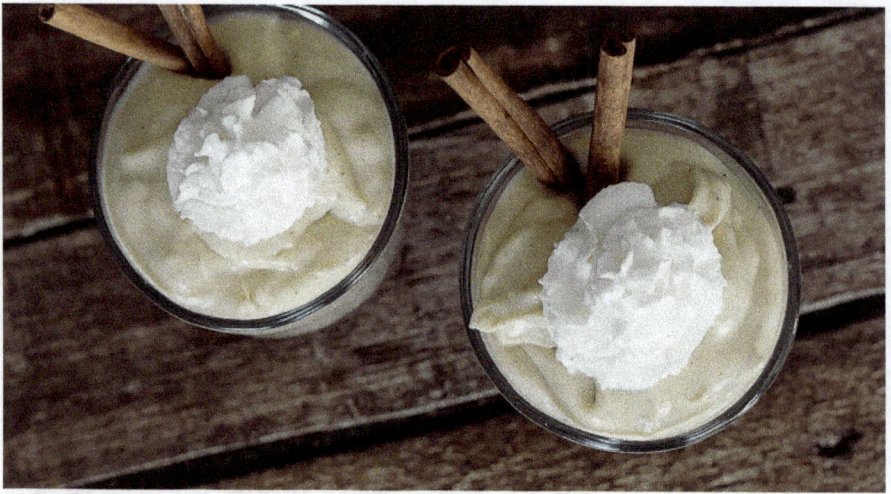

# Creamy Grapes Bowls

**Prep time:** 10 minutes I **Cooking time:** 25 minutes I
**Servings:** 4

**Ingredients:**

- 2 cups coconut milk
- ½ cup coconut cream
- ½ cup black tea
- 1 teaspoon vanilla extract
- 1 cup grapes, halved
- 1 tablespoon sugar
- 1 tablespoon maple syrup

**Directions:**

1. Heat up a pan with the coconut milk over medium heat, add the cream, the grapes and the other ingredients, bring to a simmer and cook over medium heat for 25 minutes.
2. Divide into bowls and serve cold.

**Nutrition info per serving:** calories 140, fat 4, fiber 2, carbs 6, protein 5

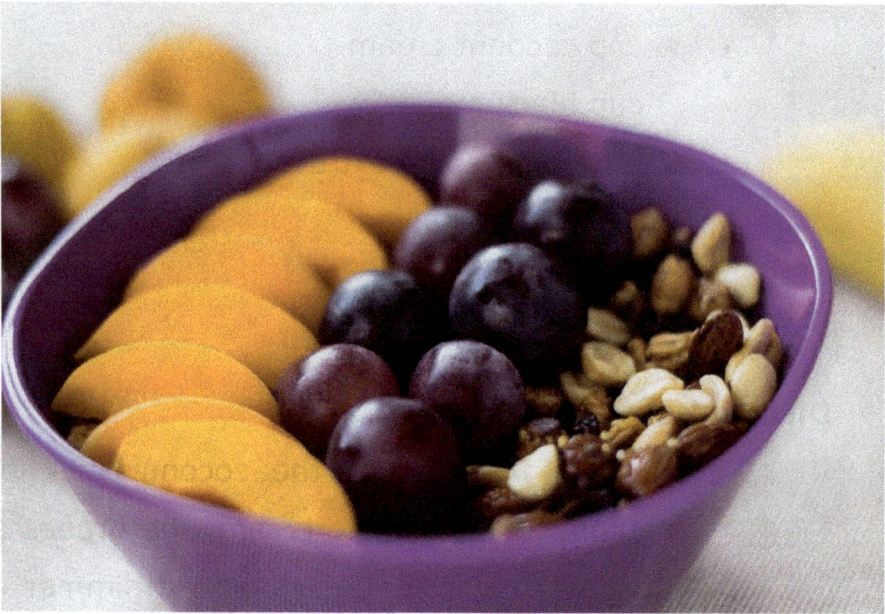

# Lemon Black Tea Cream

**Prep time:** 30 minutes I **Cooking time:** 0 minutes I
**Servings:** 4

**Ingredients:**

- 2 cups coconut cream
- ½ cup black tea, brewed
- Juice of 1 lemon
- Zest of 1 lemon, grated
- 1 teaspoon vanilla extract
- 2 tablespoons chicory root powder

**Directions:**

1. In a bowl, combine the cream with the lemon
   juice and the other ingredients, whisk, divide
   into bowls and keep in the fridge for 30 minutes
   before serving.

**Nutrition info per serving:** calories 279, fat 28.6, fiber
2.6, carbs 6.8, protein 2.8

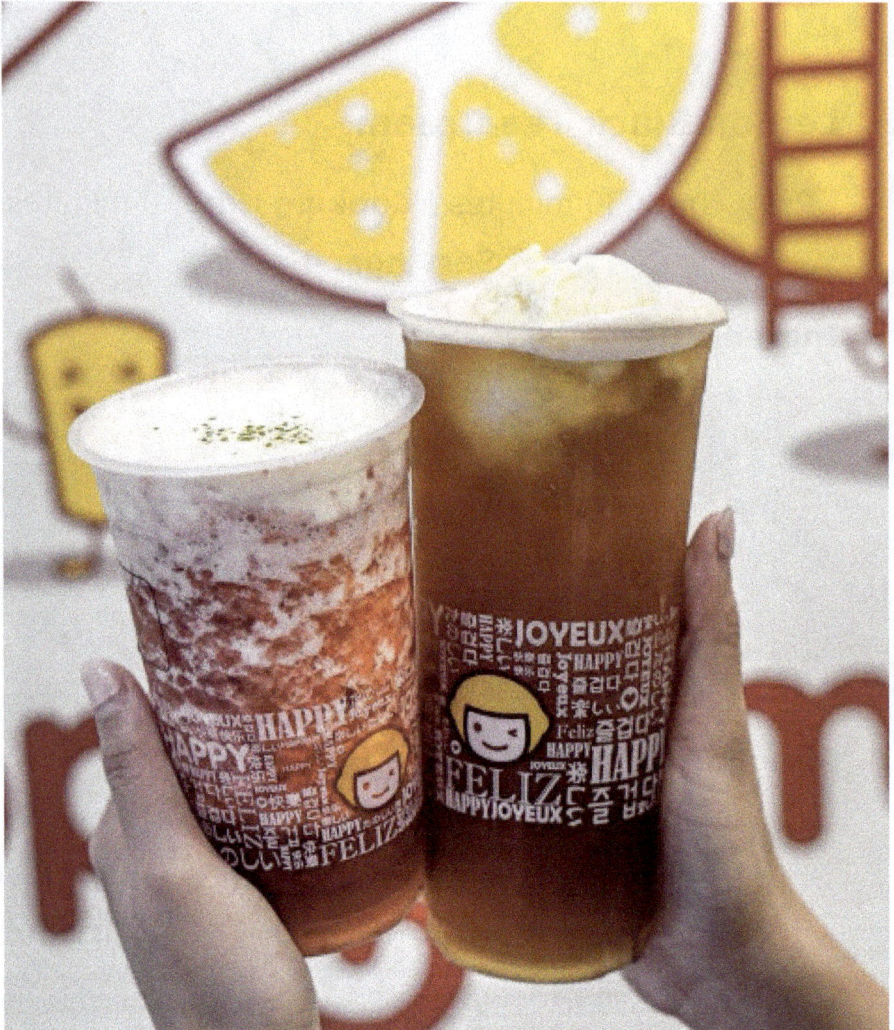

# Rice and Cantaloupe Pudding

**Prep time:** 10 minutes I **Cooking time:** 30 minutes I
**Servings:** 4

**Ingredients:**

- 2 cup coconut milk
- 1 cup black rice
- 3 tablespoons chicory root powder
- 1 small cantaloupe, peeled and chopped
- 1 teaspoon cinnamon powder

**Directions:**

1. In a pan, combine the milk with the rice and the
   other ingredients, whisk, bring to a simmer and
   cook over medium heat for 30 minutes.
2. Divide the pudding into bowls and serve.

**Nutrition info per serving:** calories 276, fat 28.6, fiber
2.6, carbs 6.7, protein 2.8

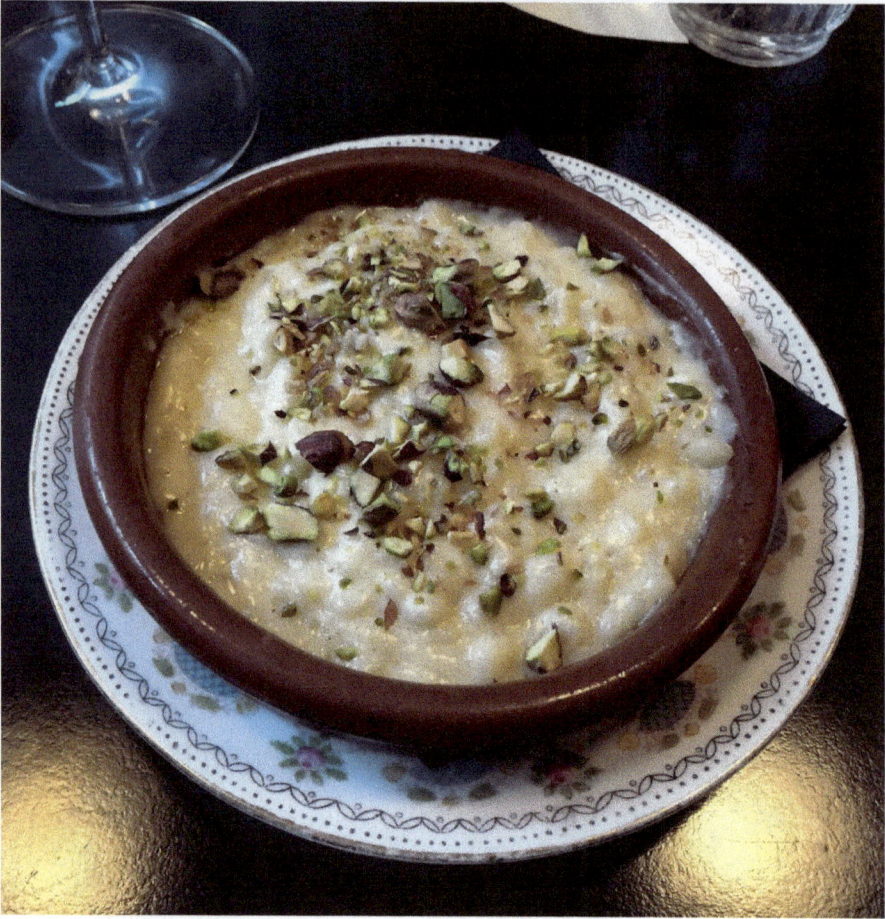

# Chocolate Nuts Mix

**Prep time:** 10 minutes I **Cooking time:** 10 minutes I
**Servings:** 6

## Ingredients:

- 2 cups coconut milk
- 1 cup coconut cream
- ¼ cup walnuts, chopped
- ½ cup dark chocolate, chopped

## Directions:

1. Put the milk in a pan, heat up over medium heat, add the cream, chocolate and the other ingredients and cook for 10 minutes stirring often.
2. Transfer this bowls and serve warm.

**Nutrition info per serving:** calories 204, fat 15, fiber 4, carbs 10, protein 5

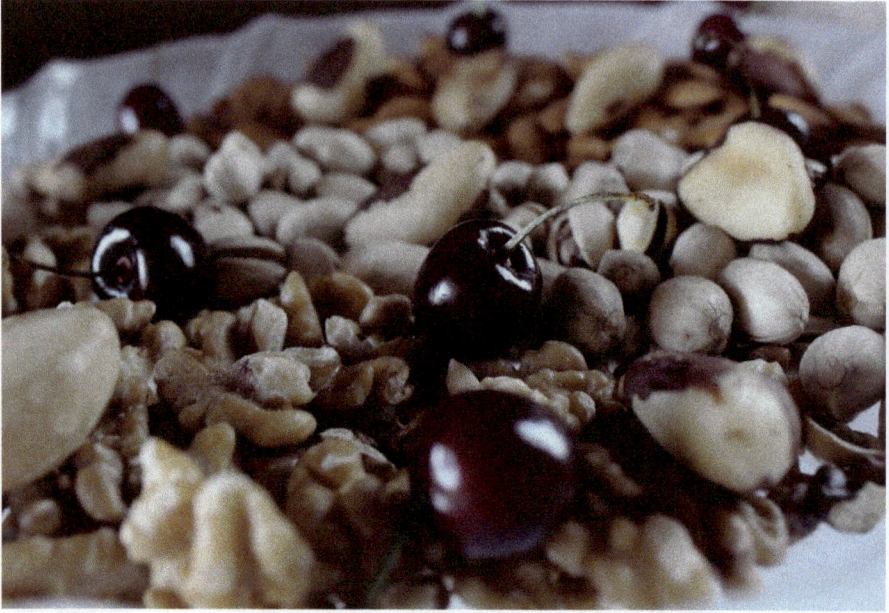

# Mixed Fruits

**Prep time:** 10 minutes I **Cooking time:** 0 minutes I
**Servings:** 4

**Ingredients:**

- 1 avocado, peeled, pitted and chopped
- 1 big banana, peeled and chopped
- 1 mango, peeled and cubed
- 1 tablespoon honey
- ½ cup grapes, halved
- 1 tablespoon lime juice
- 2 teaspoons lime zest, grated

**Directions:**

1. In a bowl, combine the avocado with the banana and the other ingredients, toss, divide into small bowls and serve.

**Nutrition info per serving:** calories 207, fat 10.3, fiber 5.8, carbs 31.1, protein 2.1

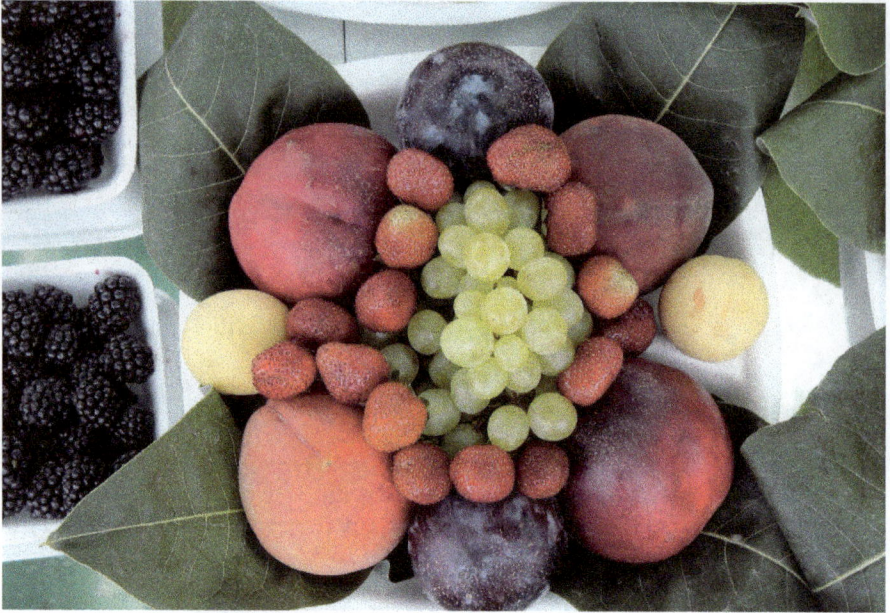

# Banana Cake

**Prep time:** 10 minutes I **Cooking time:** 30 minutes
I**Servings:** 6

## Ingredients:

- 2 tablespoons green tea powder
- 2 cups coconut milk
- 4 eggs, whisked
- 2 bananas, peeled and chopped
- 2 teaspoons vanilla extract
- 2 cups almond flour
- 1 teaspoon baking soda

## Directions:

1. In a bowl, combine the coconut milk with the green tea powder and the other ingredients, stir well, pour into a cake pan, introduce in the oven and bake at 350 degrees F for 30 minutes.
2. Slice and serve cold.

**Nutrition info per serving:** calories 490, fat 39.9, fiber 7.1, carbs 21.8, protein 14.3

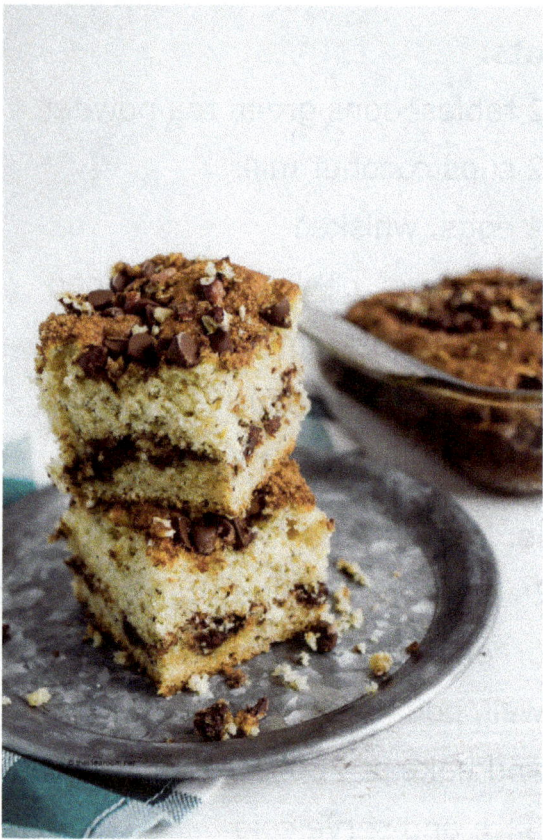

# Chia Coconut Mix

**Prep time:** 2 hours I **Cooking time:** 0 minutes I
**Servings:** 4

**Ingredients:**

- 2 cups almond milk
- 1 cup coconut cream
- 2 tablespoons chia seeds
- 2 tablespoons coconut, unsweetened and shredded
- 1 tablespoon chicory root powder
- 1 teaspoon cocoa powder

**Directions:**

1. In a bowl, combine the almond milk with the cream, chia seeds and the other ingredients, whisk well, divide into smaller bowls and keep in the fridge for 2 hours before serving.

**Nutrition info per serving:** calories 493, fat 48.2, fiber 9.2, carbs 16.6, protein 6.6

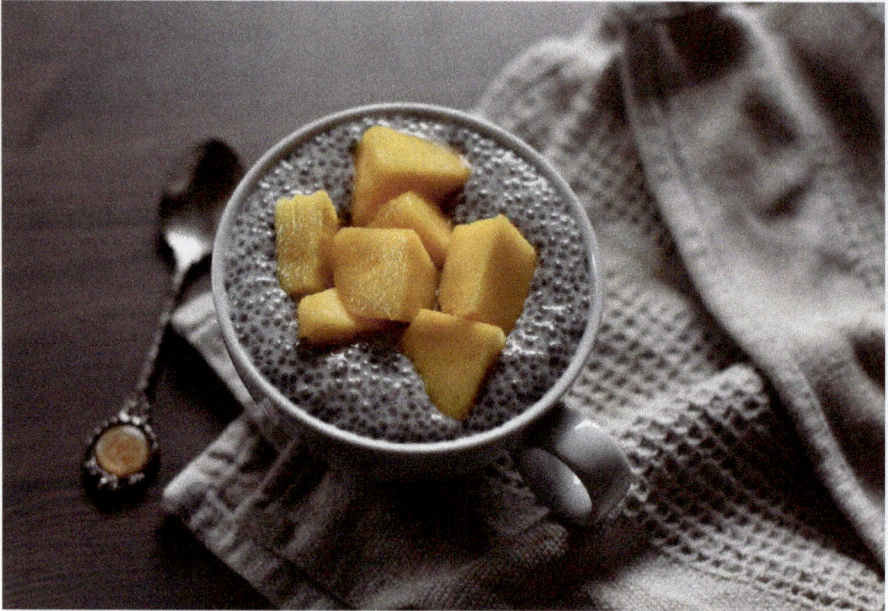

# Grapes Salad

**Prep time:** 5 minutes I **Cooking time:** 0 minutes I

**Servings:** 2

**Ingredients:**

- 1 cup cantaloupe, peeled and cubed
- 1 cup grapes, halved
- 2 tablespoons mint, chopped
- 1 tablespoon honey
- 1 teaspoon nutmeg, ground
- 1 teaspoon vanilla extract
- 1 tablespoon lemon juice

**Directions:**

1. In a bowl, combine the cantaloupe with the grapes, mint and the other ingredients, toss, divide into smaller bowls and serve.

**Nutrition info per serving:** calories 105, fat 0.8, fiber 1.8, carbs 24.4, protein 1.3

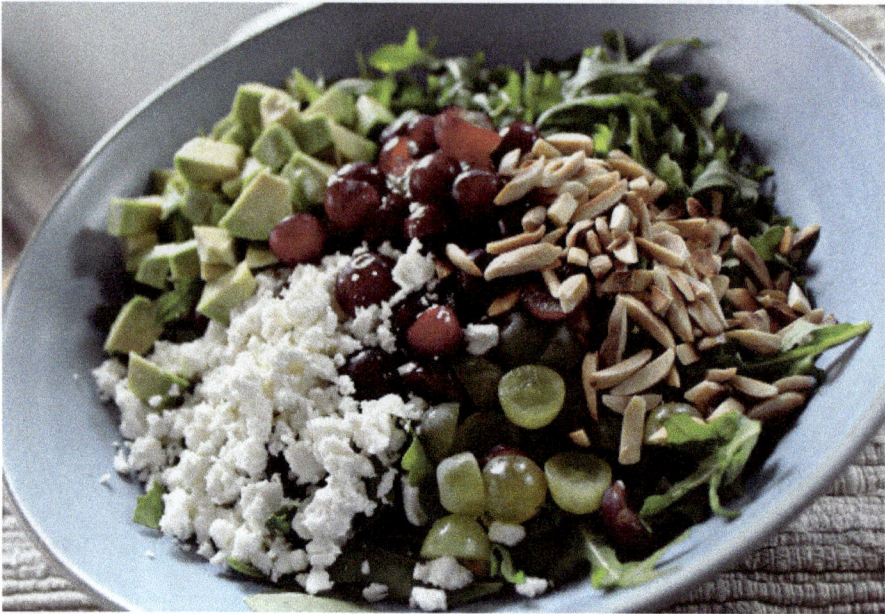

# Raspberry Bars

**Prep time:** 10 minutes I **Cooking time:** 5 minutes I
**Servings:** 12

## Ingredients:

- ½ cup coconut butter
- ½ cup coconut oil
- ½ cup raspberries, dried
- ¼ cup stevia
- ½ cup coconut, shredded

## Directions:

1. In a food processor, blend dried berries.
2. Heat a pan with butter over medium heat. Add oil, coconut, and stevia, stir, and cook for 5 minutes.
3. Pour half into a lined baking pan and spread well.
4. Add raspberry powder and spread well.
5. Top with remaining butter mixture, spread, and keep in refrigerator for a couple of hours, then cut into pieces and serve.

**Nutrition info per serving:** calories 124, fat 13.1, fiber 1.5, carbs 2.3, protein 0.5

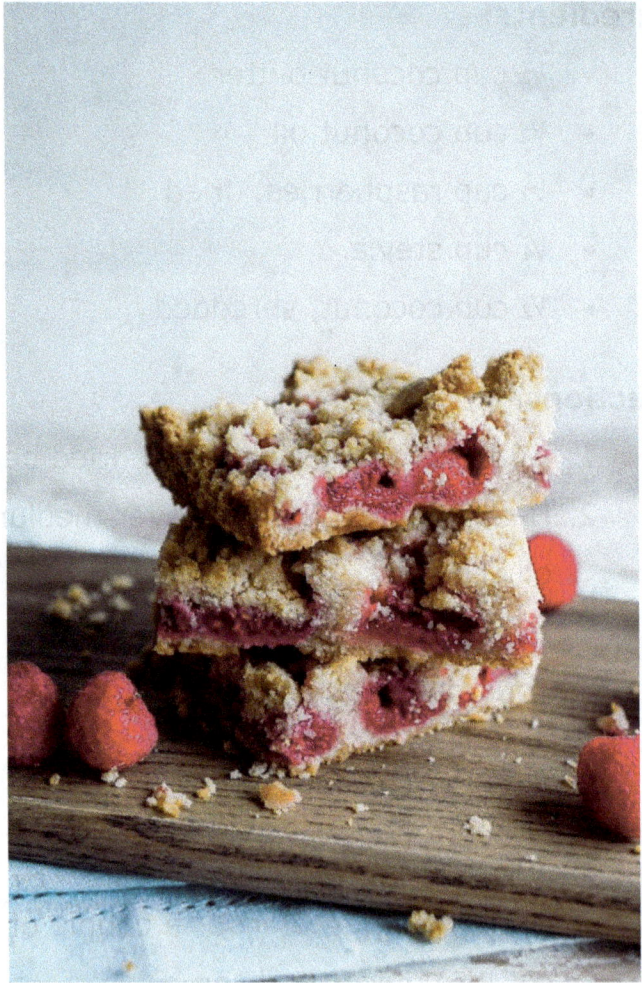

# Chocolate Balls

**Prep time:** 10 minutes I **Cooking time:** 10 minutes I
**Servings:** 12

## Ingredients:

- 10 tablespoons avocado oil
- 3 tablespoons macadamia nuts, chopped
- 2 packets stevia
- 5 tablespoons unsweetened coconut powder
- A pinch of salt

## Directions:

1. Put coconut oil in a saucepan and melt over medium heat.
2. Add stevia, salt, cocoa powder, stir well, and take off heat.
3. Spoon into a candy tray and keep in refrigerator for a couple of hours.
4. Sprinkle macadamia nuts on top and keep in the refrigerator until ready to serve.

**Nutrition info per serving:** calories 137, fat 15.2, fiber 0.2, carbs1.1, protein 0.4

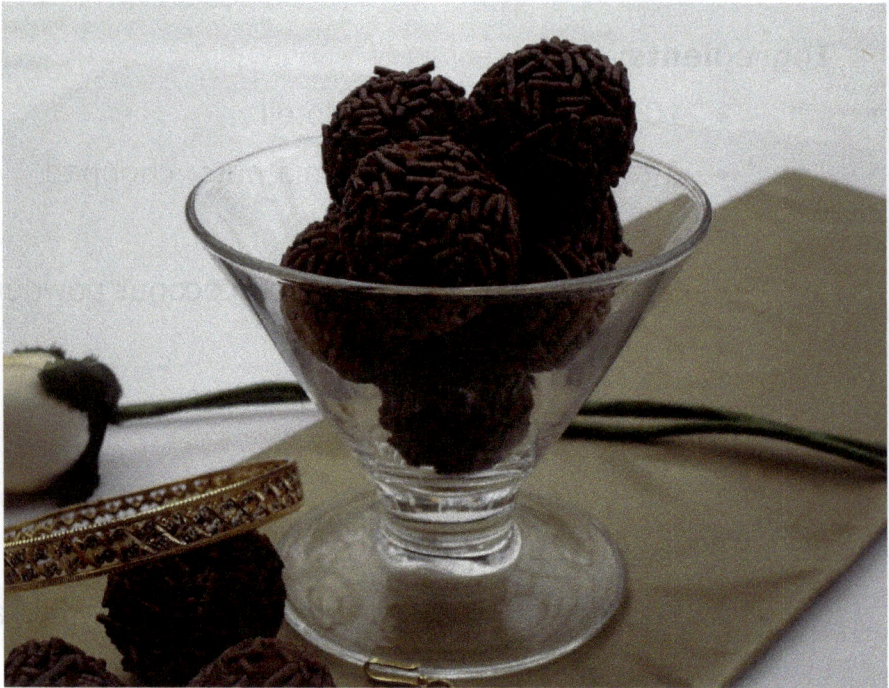

# Vanilla Jelly

**Prep. time:** 2 hours 10 minutes I **Cooking time:** 5 minutes I **Servings:** 12

**Ingredients:**

- 2 ounces gelatin
- 1 cup cold water
- 1 cup hot water
- 3 tablespoons stevia
- 2 tablespoons gelatin powder
- 1 teaspoon vanilla extract
- 1 cup heavy cream
- 1 cup boiling water

**Directions:**

1. Open gelatin packets, put gelatin powder in a bowl, add 1 cup hot water, stir until dissolved, and then mix with 1 cup cold water.

2. Pour into a lined square dish and keep in refrigerator for 1 hour. Cut into cubes and set aside.
3. In a bowl, mix erythritol with vanilla extract, 1 cup boiling water, gelatin, heavy cream, and stir well.
4. Pour half of this mix into a silicon round mold, spread gelatin cubes, and then top with rest of the gelatin.
5. Keep in the refrigerator for 1 more hour and then serve.

**Nutrition info per serving:** calories 39, fat 3.7, fiber 0, carbs 7.31, protein 1.2

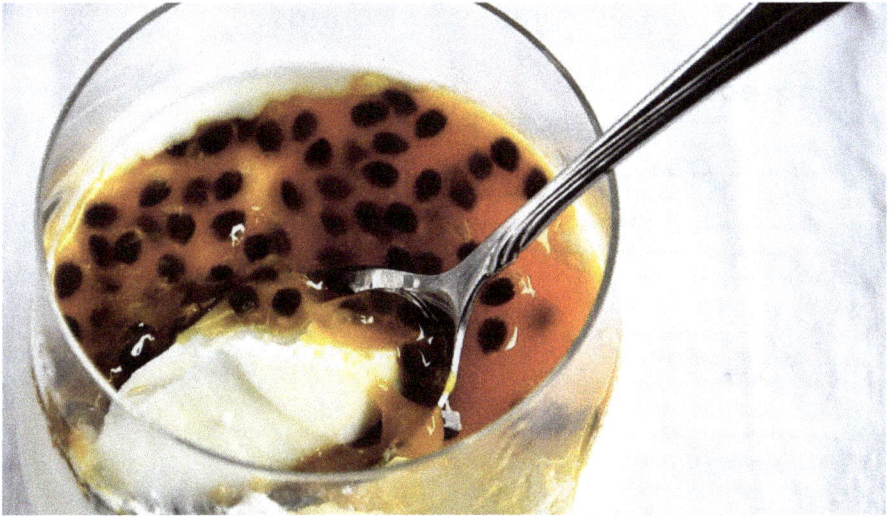

# Creamy Pie

**Prep time:** 2 hours and 10 minutes I **Cooking time:** 5 minutes I **Servings:** 12

**Ingredients:**

*For the crust:*

- 1 cup coconut, shredded
- 1 cup sunflower seeds
- ¼ cup butter
- A pinch of salt

*For the filling:*

- 1 teaspoon gelatin
- 8 ounces cream cheese
- 4 ounces strawberries
- 2 tablespoons water
- ½ tablespoon lemon juice
- ¼ teaspoon stevia
- ½ cup heavy cream
- 8 ounces strawberries, hulled, and chopped, for serving
- 16 ounces heavy cream, for serving

**Directions:**

1. In a food processor, mix sunflower seeds with coconut, a pinch of salt, butter, and stir well.
2. Put into a greased springform pan and press well on the bottom.
3. Heat a pan with water over medium heat, add gelatin, stir until it dissolves, take off heat, and set aside to cool down.
4. Add to a food processor, mix with 4 ounces strawberries, cream cheese, lemon juice, stevia, and blend well.
5. Add ½ cup heavy cream, stir well, spread over crust.
6. Top with 8 ounces strawberries, 16 ounces heavy cream and keep in the refrigerator for 2 hours before slicing and serving.

**Nutrition info per serving:** calories 201, fat 20.2, fiber 1.1, carbs 3.4, protein 2.9

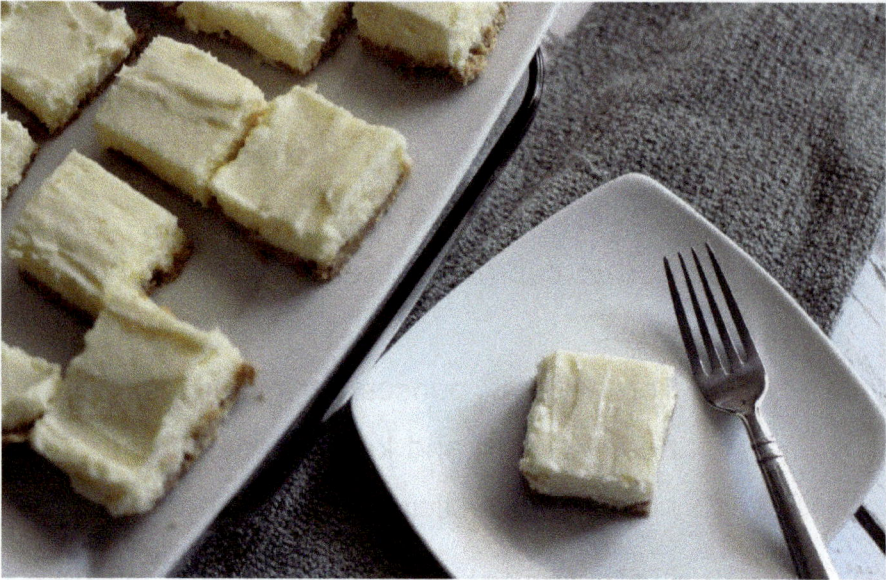

# Chocolate Cupcakes

**Prep time:** 30 minutes I **Cooking time:** 5 minutes I **Servings:** 20

**Ingredients:**

- ½ cup coconut butter
- ½ cup avocado oil
- ½ cup coconut, shredded
- 1. 5 ounces cocoa butter
- 1 ounces chocolate, unsweetened
- ¼ cup cocoa powder
- ¼ teaspoon vanilla extract
- ¼ cup swerve

**Directions:**

1. In a pan, mix coconut butter with the oil, stir, and heat up over medium heat.

2. Add coconut and stir well, take off heat, scoop into a lined muffins pan, and keep in refrigerator for 30 minutes.
3. In a bowl, mix cocoa butter with chocolate, vanilla extract, ¼ cup swerve, and stir well.
4. Place this over a bowl filled with boiling water and stir until everything is smooth.
5. Spoon over coconut cupcakes, keep in the refrigerator for 15 minutes, and then serve.

**Nutrition info per serving:** calories 201, fat 21.2, fiber 1.8, carbs 4.2, protein 0.9

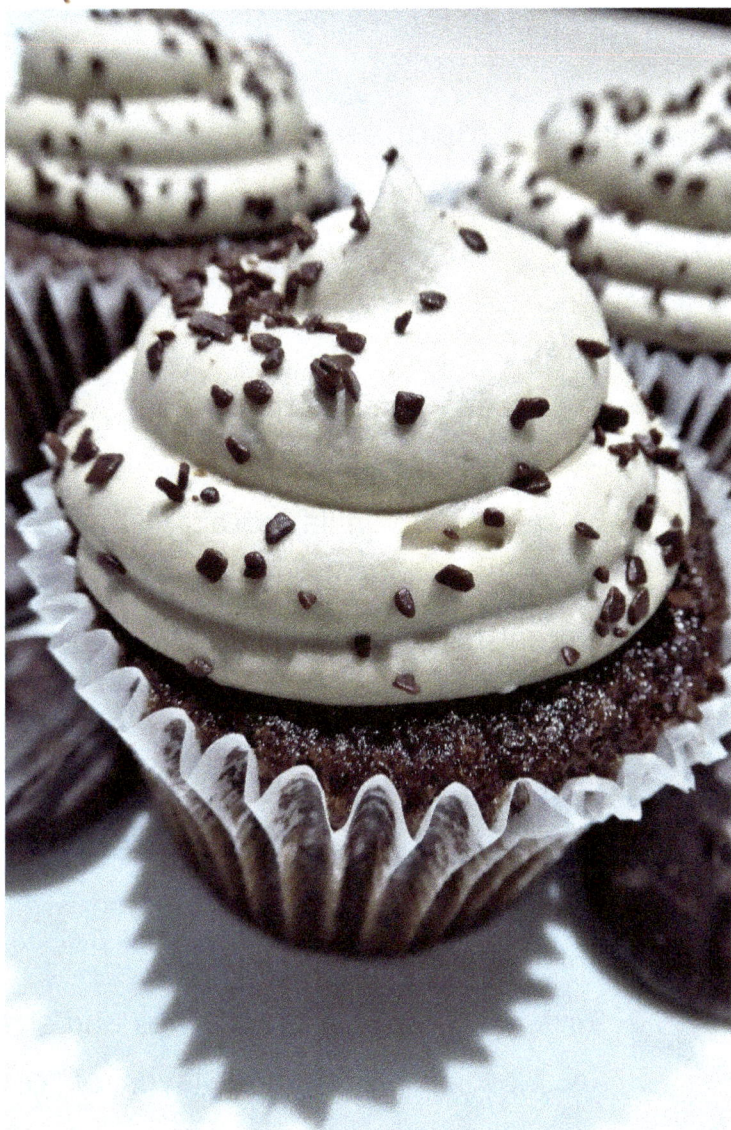

# Mascarpone Mousse

**Prep time:** 10 minutes I **Cooking time:** 0 minutes I
**Servings:** 12

**Ingredients:**

- 8 ounces mascarpone cheese
- ¾ teaspoon maple syrup
- ½ teaspoon vanilla extract
- 1 cup whipping cream
- ½ pint blueberries
- ½ pint strawberries

**Directions:**

1. In a bowl, mix whipping cream with maple syrup, mascarpone, and blend well using a mixer.
2. Arrange a layer of blueberries and strawberries in 12 glasses, then a layer of cream, and repeat. Serve cold.

**Nutrition info per serving:** calories 77, fat 5.6, fiber 0.7, carbs 2.8, protein 4.6

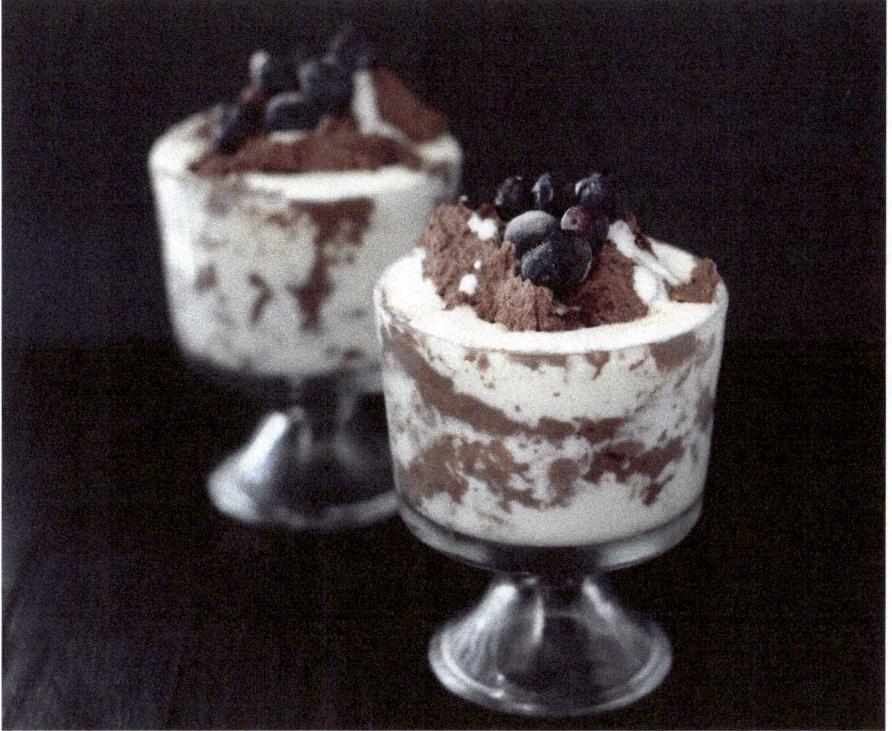

# Butter Fudge

**Prep. time:** 2 hours and 10 minutes I **Cooking time:** 2 minutes I **Servings:** 12

## Ingredients:

- 1 cup peanut butter, unsweetened
- ¼ cup almond milk
- ½ teaspoon vanilla extract
- 2 teaspoons stevia
- 1 cup coconut oil
- A pinch of salt

*For the topping:*

- 2 tablespoons avocado oil
- ¼ cup cocoa powder

## Directions:

1. In a heatproof bowl, mix peanut butter with 1 cup coconut oil, stir, and heat up in a microwave until it melts.
2. Add a pinch of salt, almond milk, stevia, stir well, and pour into a lined loaf pan.
3. Keep in refrigerator for 2 hours and then slice it.
4. In a bowl, mix 2 tablespoons avocado oil with cocoa powder, and stir well.
5. Drizzle sauce over the peanut butter fudge and serve.

**Nutrition info per serving:** calories 312, fat 31.9, fiber 1.9, carbs 6.3, protein 5.8

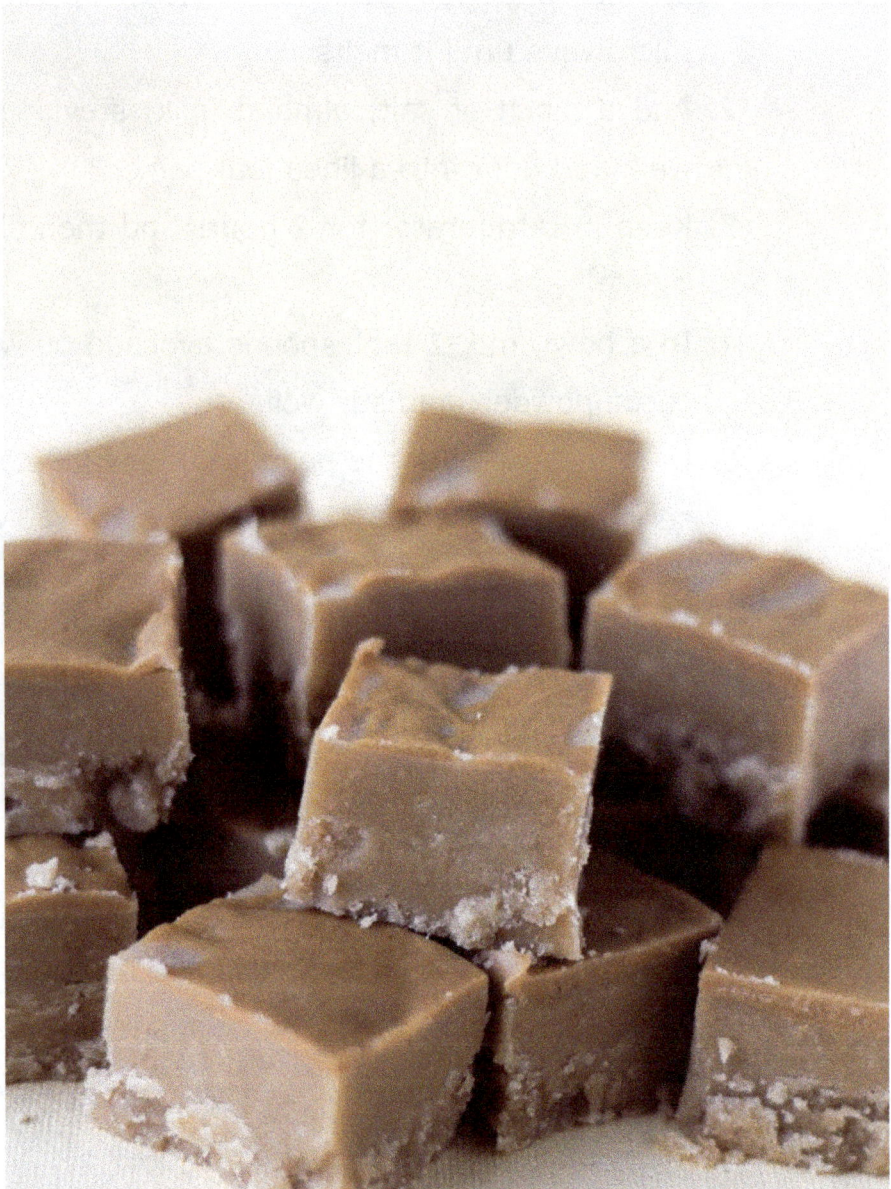

# Cream Cheese Brownies

**Prep time:** 10 minutes I **Cooking time:** 20 minutes I
**Servings:** 12

## Ingredients:

- 6 ounces avocado oil
- 6 eggs
- 3 ounces cocoa powder
- 2 teaspoons vanilla extract
- ½ teaspoon baking powder
- 4 ounces cream cheese

## Directions:

1. In a blender, mix eggs with avocado oil, cocoa powder, baking powder, vanilla extract, cream cheese, and stir using a mixer.
2. Pour into a lined baking dish, place in an oven at 350ºF and bake for 20 minutes.
3. Cool then slice into rectangle pieces, and serve.

**Nutrition info per serving:** calories 202, fat 20.6, fiber 2.1, carbs 4.3, protein 4.8

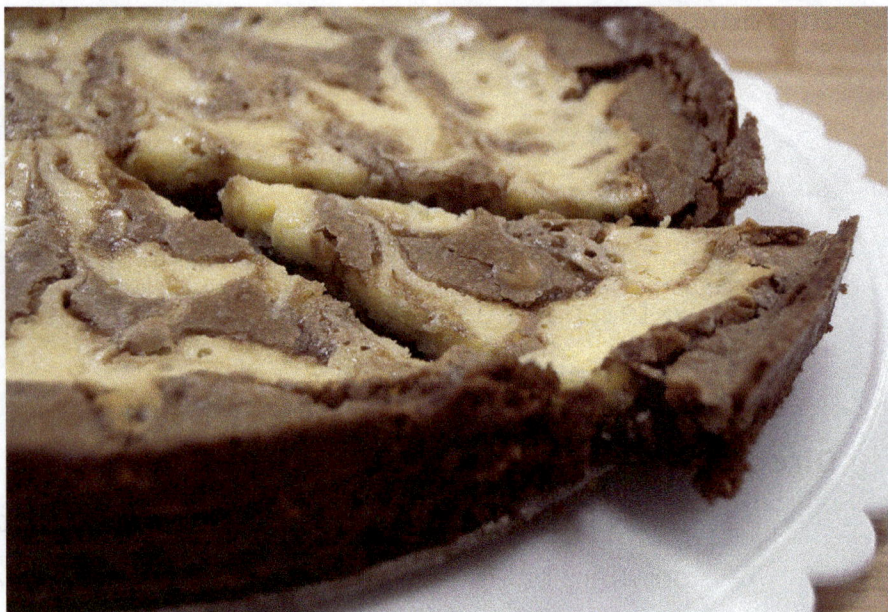

# Cocoa Almond and Avocado Pudding

**Prep time:** 50 minutes I **Cooking time:** 5 minutes I
**Servings:** 2

**Ingredients:**

- 2 tablespoons water
- 1 tablespoon gelatin
- 1 avocado, peeled, pitted and mashed
- ½ cup almonds, crushed
- 2 tablespoons cocoa powder
- 1 cup coconut milk

**Directions:**

1. Heat a pan with coconut milk over medium heat, add other ingredients except the gelatin and water, and stir well.
2. In a bowl, mix gelatin with water, stir well, and add to pan.
3. Divide into ramekins, and keep in refrigerator for 45 minutes. Serve cold.

**Nutrition info per serving:** calories 300, fat 29.3, fiber 4.3, carbs 9.6, protein 6.7

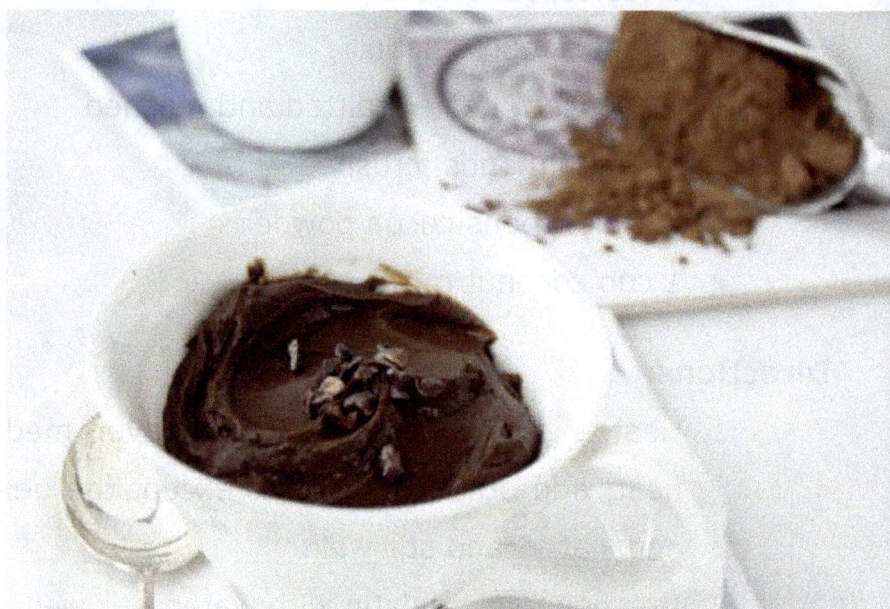

# Walnut Parfaits

**Prep time:** 10 minutes I **Cooking time:** 0 minutes I
**Servings:** 4

**Ingredients:**

- 14 ounces coconut milk
- 1 teaspoon vanilla extract
- 4 ounces mixed berries
- 2 tablespoons walnuts, chopped

**Directions:**

1. In a bowl, mix coconut milk with vanilla extract, and whisk using a mixer.
2. In another bowl, mix berries with walnuts and stir.
3. Spoon half of vanilla coconut mixture into 4 jars, add a layer of berries, and top with rest of the vanilla mixture.
4. Top with berries and walnuts mixture, place in the refrigerator to chill before serving.

**Nutrition info per serving:** calories 272, fat 26.1, fiber 3.5, carbs 9.5, protein 3.4

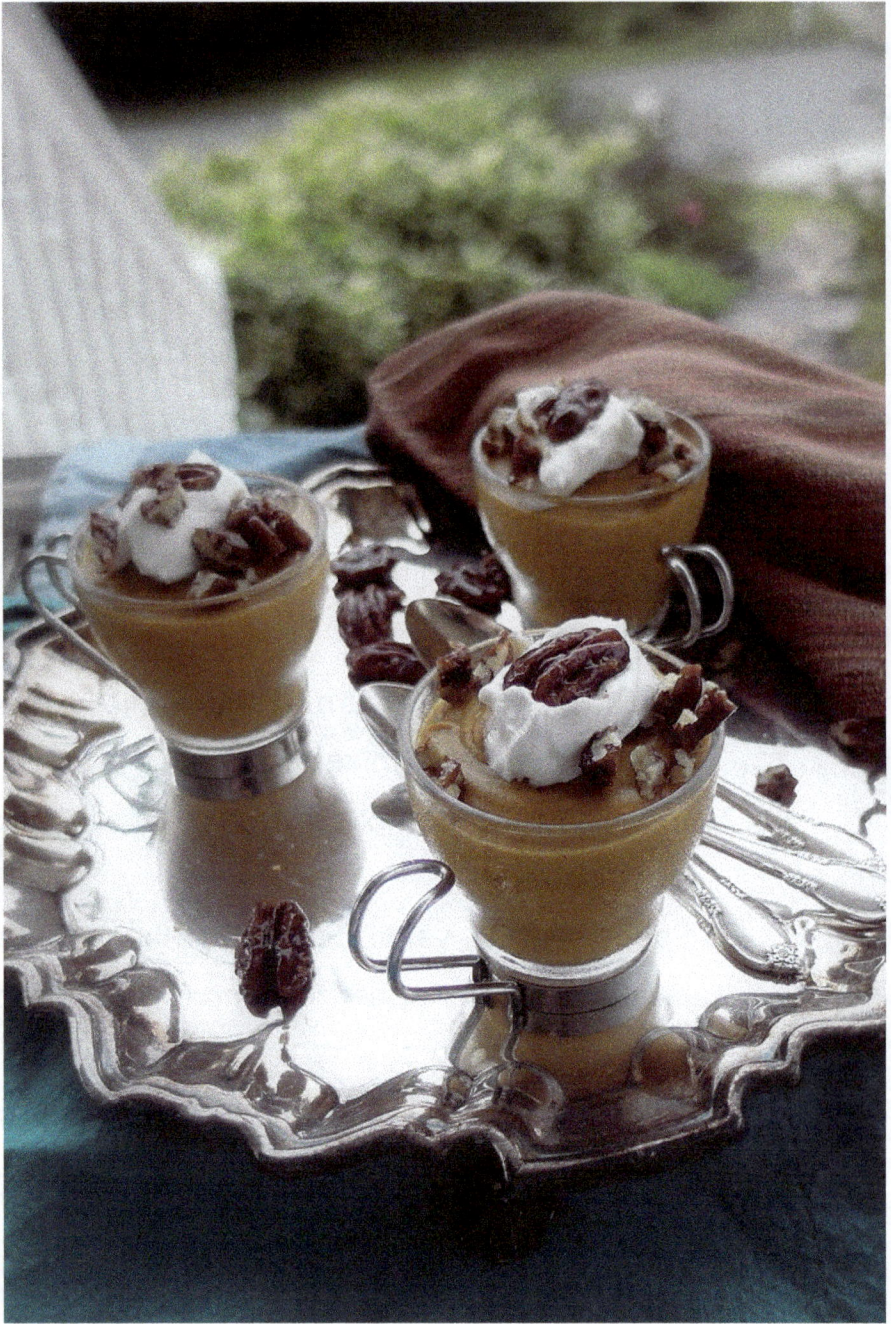